# CONDITIONING FOR A PURPOSE

HOW TO BECOME PHYSICALLY FIT
FOR SPORTS AND ATHLETICS

edited by

## James A. Peterson, Ph.D.

Leisure Press
P.O. Box 3
West Point, N.Y. 10996

*A publication of Leisure Press.*
*P.O. Box 3, West Point, N.Y. 10996*
*Copyright © 1977 by James A. Peterson*
*All rights reserved. Printed in the U.S.A.*

*Library of Congress Catalog Card No. 76-62811*
*ISBN 0-918438-01-2*

**Unless otherwise noted, credit**
**for all photographs should be**
**given to *U.S. Army Photographs***

**Cover design by Lanny Somese**

# TABLE OF CONTENTS

PREFACE . . . . . . . . . . . . . . . . . . . . . . . . . . . . . . . . . . . . . . . . . . . . . 4

PART I.   FITNESS PRINCIPLES
1. Physical Fitness: Myths and Realities . . . . . . . . . . . . . . . . . . . . .   5
2. The Human Machine. . . . . . . . . . . . . . . . . . . . . . . . . . . . . . . . . .  14
3. Strength Training: Fundamentals and Techniques. . . . . . . . . . . .  28
4. Organizing a Strength Training Program. . . . . . . . . . . . . . . . . . .  43
5. Free Weight Exercises . . . . . . . . . . . . . . . . . . . . . . . . . . . . . . . . .  60
6. Nautilus Training. . . . . . . . . . . . . . . . . . . . . . . . . . . . . . . . . . . . . 107
7. Project Total Conditioning . . . . . . . . . . . . . . . . . . . . . . . . . . . . . 133
8. Running . . . . . . . . . . . . . . . . . . . . . . . . . . . . . . . . . . . . . . . . . . . . 160
9. Women and Athletics . . . . . . . . . . . . . . . . . . . . . . . . . . . . . . . . . 173
10. Nutrition and Athletics . . . . . . . . . . . . . . . . . . . . . . . . . . . . . . . . 183
11. Injury Prevention and Treatment. . . . . . . . . . . . . . . . . . . . . . . . . 192
12. Muscle Tonus Exercises. . . . . . . . . . . . . . . . . . . . . . . . . . . . . . . . 222
13. Program Planning . . . . . . . . . . . . . . . . . . . . . . . . . . . . . . . . . . . . 229

PART II.   CONDITIONING PROGRAMS FOR SELECTED SPORTS
14. Baseball. . . . . . . . . . . . . 252
15. Basketball . . . . . . . . . . . 258
16. Bowling . . . . . . . . . . . . . 264
17. Boxing . . . . . . . . . . . . . . 267
18. Field Hockey. . . . . . . . . 271
19. Football. . . . . . . . . . . . . 275
20. Golf . . . . . . . . . . . . . . . . 280
21. Gymnastics . . . . . . . . . . 284
22. Handball . . . . . . . . . . . . 289
23. Ice Hockey . . . . . . . . . . 293
24. Judo. . . . . . . . . . . . . . . . 298
25. Lacrosse  . . . . . . . . . . 302
26. Racquetball . . . . . . . . 306
27. Rugby . . . . . . . . . . . . . 311
28. Skiing. . . . . . . . . . . . . . 319
29. Soccer . . . . . . . . . . . . . 323
30. Swimming . . . . . . . . . . 327
31. Team Handball. . . . . . . 331
32. Tennis . . . . . . . . . . . . . 335
33. Track and Field. . . . . . . 339
34. Volleyball . . . . . . . . . . . 343
35. Wrestling. . . . . . . . . . . . 349

# PREFACE

Whether it is better to exercise **this way** or **that way** has been debated for years. Unfortunately, much of the dialogue concerning exercise has been based on unfounded superstitions and intuitions. **Conditioning for a Purpose** discredits the mythology surrounding physical fitness.

Part I of **Conditioning for a Purpose** examines the basic concepts and foundations of fitness training. Part II offers individualized programs for twenty-two separate sports. These programs are a must for **coaches** and **athletes** at all levels of competition.

The book is a compendium of the efforts of the Personal Conditioning Committee of the Office of Physical Education, United States Military Academy, West Point. Written by faculty from an institution where personal fitness maintenance is an integral part of the curriculum, **Conditioning for a Purpose** is designed for everyone interested in improving his/her athletic performance.

James A. Peterson, Ph.D.
Editor

# CHAPTER 1
## Physical Fitness: Myths and Realities

James A. Peterson, Ph.D.

What factors affect athletic performance?
What are the basic steps involved in developing a conditioning program
to improve athletic performance?
What is physical fitness?
What are the qualities basic to physical fitness?
What are the basic motor ability functions?
What are the two most important principles of conditioning?

Athletes should work out two or three hours a day if they want to achieve maximum levels of personal fitness...Athletes who lift weights become muscle bound...When athletes stop competing, their muscles turn to fat...Athletes should avoid water during training sessions... Protein supplements aid strength development...Women athletes who lift weights develop massive muscles and masculine traits...Heat is the best treatment for muscle pulls and strains...Steak should be an integral part of the menu for the pre-competition meal...Strength training cannot improve cardio-respiratory fitness...

The aforementioned are but a few of the seemingly endless list of myths, superstitions, and practices incorporated into many conditioning programs. Although the origins of these fantasies are varied, such practices and idiosynchronacies have at least one commonality — THEY ARE COUNTERPRODUCTIVE TO THE MOST EFFECTIVE METHODS OF CONDITIONING!

For athletes who seek to improve their level of fitness (and subsequently, their level of athletic performance), the task is obvious— base their conditioning program on sound, scientific principles. Only by separating fact from intuition and fiction will the athlete be able to develop the most effective personal conditioning program. Although there are few absolutes in conditioning, the body of knowledge related to conditioning for athletics is constantly expanding. Many coaches and athletes are either too apathetic to modify outdated training practices of the past or simply do not keep abreast of new developments in physical conditioning. Unfortunately, they are shortchanging their athletes and themselves by ot taking advantage of the most up-to-date research-proven methods for sports conditioning and training.

**Conditioning for a Purpose** provides a framework for both the coach and the athlete who are seeking a feasible, effective conditioning program which will improve athletic performance. Conditioning guidelines are presented. Questions are answered. Programs are suggested. The reader is urged to remember, however, that conditioning programs are, by nature, heterogeneous. As a result, each reader must apply the information presented in this book to his own strengths, weaknesses, and tolerances.

## WHAT FACTORS AFFECT ATHLETIC PERFORMANCE?

The factors which affect the performance of an athlete can collectively be grouped into two broad categories: external and internal. The **external factors** include those items over which the athlete frequently has only limited (if any) control — such as climate, facilities, abilities of his opponents, skills of his teammates, etc. The **internal factors**, on the other hand, are subject 'to substantial personal influence. Frequently referred to in the literature under a wide variety of designations and terms, the internal factors can be grouped into three general divisions: (1) physical fitness level; (2) motor ability; and (3) mental toughness. The motor ability of an athlete is his capacity to perform particular motor functions — e.g. coordination and balance. The third and final category of internal factors — mental toughness — reflects the totality of an athlete's mental commitment to perform at his highest possible level. It includes such interrelated intangibles as positive attitudes, self-discipline, high motivation, and perserverance.

## WHAT ARE THE BASIC STEPS INVOLVED IN DEVELOPING A CONDITIONING PROGRAM TO IMPROVE ATHLETIC PERFORMANCE?

Listing the possible actions involved in improving an athlete's level of "mental toughness" would require several volumes in addition to this text. **Conditioning for a Purpose** examines the considerations attendant to improving the physical fitness level of an athlete. Improvement in motor ability is also discussed to the extent that an individual's motor skills are at least partially dependent on his level of physical fitness.

Having mentally committed himself to improving his level of athletic performance, the athlete should proceed by undertaking the following steps:

(1) Identify the full range of specific activities involved in the sport or position of interest. For example, an offensive lineman in tackle football should be able to block for a run, pull for a block, block for a pass, etc.

(2) Identify the major muscles involved in the specific activities

attendant to a sport. For example, the trapezius muscle is one of the primary muscles involved in passing a football. (Chapter 4 provides an inclusive listing of the muscles of the body and their function during sports activity.)

(3) Identify the quality or component of fitness required to perform the activities involved in a sport. For example, sufficient leg strength is one of the requirements for kicking a football.

(4) Based upon the information obtained in steps 1-3, develop a program which is tailored to increase his capability to perform in the sport. Obviously, this is a two-fold task: correctly analyzing the sports physical requirements and then selecting activities which will improve the athlete's capacity to meet the requirements.

## WHAT IS PHYSICAL FITNESS?

Given sufficient time and energy, an individual could probably locate more than 100 similar, yet distinct, definitions of "physical fitness" in the literature. Because of its strong correlation, with both common sense and the existing body of knowledge concerning personal conditioning, the following definition has been adopted for this book:

"Physical fitness is the individual capacity to engage in physical activities of a reasonably vigorous nature."

Such a definition implies that being physically fit involves more than the capacity to carry out normal, every-day physically non-demanding tasks. In addition, no mention is made of motor skills. An individual could, as a matter of course, be reasonably physically fit and yet be a below-average performer in a given sport because he lacks the requisite motor ability or the necessary mental toughness.

## WHAT ARE THE QUALITIES BASIC TO PHYSICAL FITNESS?

Depending upon whether or not muscular fitness is viewed as being one or two of the primary aspects of fitness, there are four (perhaps five) qualities basic to physical fitness.

1. **Cardiovascular Fitness** is that aspect of fitness which enables an individual to engage in strenuous activity for extended periods of time. Dependent upon the combined efficiency of the heart, circulatory vessels, and lungs, cardiovascular fitness is an integral factor in an athlete's performance in sports which involve the use of much of the body's large musculature (e.g. soccer, lacrosse and football). The reason for this is that sports in which the large

muscles of the body are extensively utilized require that the heart, lungs, and circulatory vessels operate at greater than usual levels of efficiency. When an athlete's circulatory and respiratory systems fail to meet the cardiovascular demands of the sport, performance suffers.

2. **Muscular Fitness** is that quality of fitness which enables an individual to engage in activities requiring greater-than-normal levels of muscular development. The literature is equivocal, however, concerning the "nature" of muscular development. Some individuals claim that such development is inclusive in that it encompasses both of the two basic applications of muscular work — endurance and force. Other individuals argue that although the ability to persist in a localized muscle group activity (endurance) and the ability to exert force (strength) are interrelated, the two factors are separate, distinct qualities of fitness. "Muscular endurance" can be defined as that aspect of muscular fitness which enables an athlete to engage in localized muscle group activities (e.g. hitting a ceiling shot in handball and pitching a baseball) for an extended period of time with relative, comparable effectiveness. "Muscular strength" is the maximum amount of force that can be exerted by a muscle or muscle group. It is specific to a given muscle or muscle group and is related to the nature of the resistance — that is, whether it is movable (dynamic or isotonic) or fixed (isometric).

3. **Flexibility** is the functional capacity of a joint to move through a normal range of motion. It is specific to given joints and is dependent primarily on the musculature surrounding a joint. Figures 1-1 and 1-2 illustrate the "normal" range of motion for the majority of the joints in the body. Both common sense and recent research lend credence to the importance of flexibility in all forms of sport. A dramatic illustration of the importance of flexibility in sports is provided in Figure 1-3.

4. **Body Composition** is an indicator of the amount of fat stored in the body. It is an important quality of fitness for the athlete because there is considerable evidence that excess fat stored in the body limits athlete's performance. Normal values of fat as a percentage of total body weight vary between men and women. The **upper** limit of "normal" for men is 18% and for women 28%. There are no established minimal levels for body fat. If an athlete receives adequate nutrition, it is not possible to be **too** lean. Different sports require varying proportions of body fat for maximum performance. A minimum amount of fat is desirable for

8

participants in such activities as distance running, high jumping and gymnastics. Athletes in those sports are hindered by added weight. Distance swimmers, on the other hand, are aided by a certain amount of fat distributed near the skin surface to diminish the heat loss to water.

## WHAT ARE THE BASIC MOTOR ABILITY FUNCTIONS?

Motor ability is one of the three major groupings of internal factors which affect athletic performance. As used in this text, motor ability is defined as the collective capability to perform selected motor functions. These functions play a critical role in athletic performance. For many athletes, the existence of high levels of ability of these motor functions frequently make the difference between being a champion or an also-ran. In general, individual ability in these functions is affected by a variety of factors — two of which can, to some extent, be influenced by a person's own efforts: (1) physical fitness (by conditioning); and (2) neuromuscular efficiency (by practicing the skill).

The basic motor functions are defined as follows:

**Agility** — is the ability to change directions rapidly and effectively while moving at a high rate of speed.

**Balance** — is the ability of an individual to maintain a specific body position while either stationary or moving.

**Coordination** — is the smooth, desired flow of movement in the execution of a motor task. Forceful and explosive movements are blended with accurate and less forceful movements to achieve purposeful movement.

**Kinesthetic sense** — is an individual's ability to be aware of the positions of various parts of the body. It is particularly important in athletics.

**Movement time** — is the time required to move **part** of the body from one point to another.

**Reaction time** — is the time required for an individual to initiate a response to a specific stimulus.

**Response time** — is movement time plus reaction time.

**Speed** — is the amount of time required to move the **entire** body from one place to another.

## WHAT ARE THE TWO MOST IMPORTANT PRINCIPLES OF CONDITIONING?

(1) **Demand** expresses the principle that in order for substantial im-

## Figure 1-1. Range of motion for fundamental movements: anterior view.

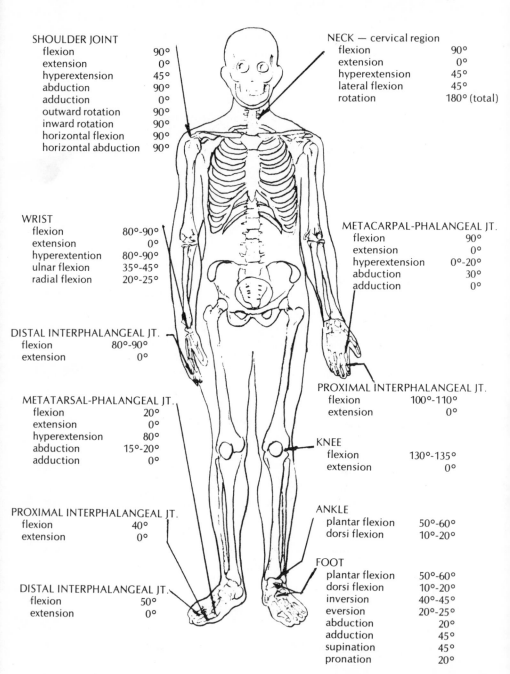

SHOULDER JOINT
| | |
|---|---|
| flexion | 90° |
| extension | 0° |
| hyperextension | 45° |
| abduction | 90° |
| adduction | 0° |
| outward rotation | 90° |
| inward rotation | 90° |
| horizontal flexion | 90° |
| horizontal abduction | 90° |

NECK — cervical region
| | |
|---|---|
| flexion | 90° |
| extension | 0° |
| hyperextension | 45° |
| lateral flexion | 45° |
| rotation | 180° (total) |

WRIST
| | |
|---|---|
| flexion | 80°-90° |
| extension | 0° |
| hyperextention | 80°-90° |
| ulnar flexion | 35°-45° |
| radial flexion | 20°-25° |

METACARPAL-PHALANGEAL JT.
| | |
|---|---|
| flexion | 90° |
| extension | 0° |
| hyperextension | 0°-20° |
| abduction | 30° |
| adduction | 0° |

DISTAL INTERPHALANGEAL JT.
| | |
|---|---|
| flexion | 80°-90° |
| extension | 0° |

METATARSAL-PHALANGEAL JT.
| | |
|---|---|
| flexion | 20° |
| extension | 0° |
| hyperextension | 80° |
| abduction | 15°-20° |
| adduction | 0° |

PROXIMAL INTERPHALANGEAL JT.
| | |
|---|---|
| flexion | 100°-110° |
| extension | 0° |

KNEE
| | |
|---|---|
| flexion | 130°-135° |
| extension | 0° |

PROXIMAL INTERPHALANGEAL JT.
| | |
|---|---|
| flexion | 40° |
| extension | 0° |

ANKLE
| | |
|---|---|
| plantar flexion | 50°-60° |
| dorsi flexion | 10°-20° |

DISTAL INTERPHALANGEAL JT.
| | |
|---|---|
| flexion | 50° |
| extension | 0° |

FOOT
| | |
|---|---|
| plantar flexion | 50°-60° |
| dorsi flexion | 10°-20° |
| inversion | 40°-45° |
| eversion | 20°-25° |
| abduction | 20° |
| adduction | 45° |
| supination | 45° |
| pronation | 20° |

## Figure 1-2. Range of motion for fundamental movements: posterior view.

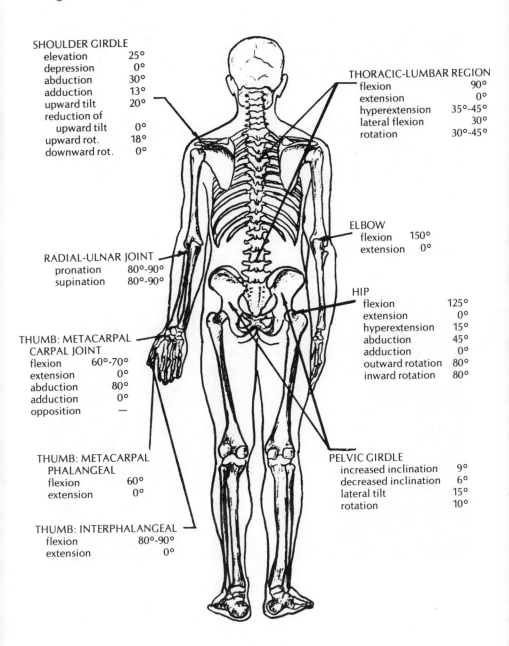

**SHOULDER GIRDLE**
| | |
|---|---|
| elevation | 25° |
| depression | 0° |
| abduction | 30° |
| adduction | 13° |
| upward tilt | 20° |
| reduction of | |
| upward tilt | 0° |
| upward rot. | 18° |
| downward rot. | 0° |

**THORACIC-LUMBAR REGION**
| | |
|---|---|
| flexion | 90° |
| extension | 0° |
| hyperextension | 35°-45° |
| lateral flexion | 30° |
| rotation | 30°-45° |

**ELBOW**
| | |
|---|---|
| flexion | 150° |
| extension | 0° |

**RADIAL-ULNAR JOINT**
| | |
|---|---|
| pronation | 80°-90° |
| supination | 80°-90° |

**HIP**
| | |
|---|---|
| flexion | 125° |
| extension | 0° |
| hyperextension | 15° |
| abduction | 45° |
| adduction | 0° |
| outward rotation | 80° |
| inward rotation | 80° |

**THUMB: METACARPAL CARPAL JOINT**
| | |
|---|---|
| flexion | 60°-70° |
| extension | 0° |
| abduction | 80° |
| adduction | 0° |
| opposition | — |

**THUMB: METACARPAL PHALANGEAL**
| | |
|---|---|
| flexion | 60° |
| extension | 0° |

**PELVIC GIRDLE**
| | |
|---|---|
| increased inclination | 9° |
| decreased inclination | 6° |
| lateral tilt | 15° |
| rotation | 10° |

**THUMB: INTERPHALANGEAL**
| | |
|---|---|
| flexion | 80°-90° |
| extension | 0° |

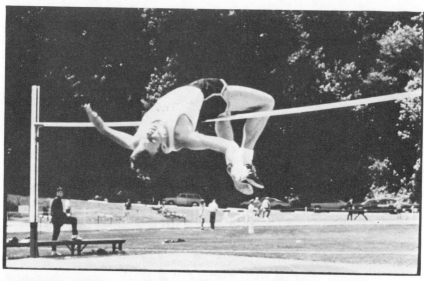

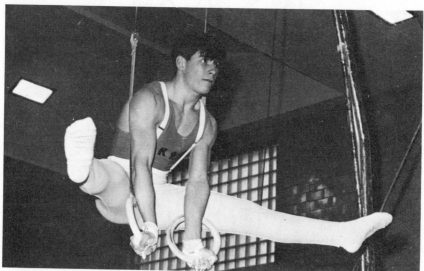

Figure 1-3. Flexibility is an important factor in many sports.

provement to occur in a system of the body or in a quality of physical fitness, the system must be stressed beyond its normal limits. If a demand is not placed on a system, no improvement will occur in that system. For example, an athlete who can curl 80# will not improve the strength of his biceps muscle by curling 50#. By the same token, a five minute miler will not break the five-minute barrier by practicing six-minute miles. Physiological responses occur within the body because of a particular need for that response.

(2) **Specificity** expresses the principle that "you get what you work for". For the athlete who wishes to improve a specific skill or capability, the best method is to practice that activity. In other words, nothing replaces the activity itself for the athlete who wishes to improve his ability to perform the activity. This is not to insinuate, however, that no benefit can be derived from non-specific acts of personal conditioning.

# CHAPTER 2
## The Human Machine

Robert M. Hensler
Captain, Infantry

A basic overview of exercise physiology
Role of foodstuffs in exercise
Applications for training
Role of oxygen in energy production and work
Contributions of energy systems to athletic performance
Stress adaptation
Cardiorespiratory system
Adaptations to exercise
Aerobic training
Anaerobic training

What causes the painful fatigue that a sprinter experiences toward the end of a 400 meter dash, or the exhaustion of a wrestler after an all out session on the mat? What types of training programs might help these athletes better their performance? These questions and more, relating to conditioning and sports fitness, will be answered in this chapter.

Frequently, a gap exists between scientific fact and actual practice, in organized athletics as well as in personal conditioning programs. By presenting an overview of exercise physiology, this chapter examines the scientific basis underlying sports training and hopefully provides the reader with some "why" as well as the "how" of getting in shape.

ROLE OF FOODSTUFFS IN EXERCISE

The human body may be compared to a machine. Some form of raw material is taken in where it is worked upon or altered and a product is produced. Foodstuffs are the raw materials of the body. Once ingested, internal processes alter the food so that it may be available for use as energy. Muscular contraction results then as work output.

The body's principal fuels are fats and carbohydrates. Fat provides for the most efficient storage of energy as it has more than twice the energy potential as an equal quantity of carbohydrates. Since the average male carries about 10-18% of his body weight as fat and the average female around 23% of her weight as fat, the human body has roughly 40-60% more energy stored as fat than carbohydrate. It is no surprise then that the body primarily burns fat for energy, particularly during long duration, low intensity activities. Routine daily tasks such as office work, resting, and walking are accomplished at the expense of fats. Jogging and most forms of manual labor done continuously are also supported partially by energy from fats.

Unfortunately the use of fat is limited as a source of energy. Because it is chemically more complex and contains less oxygen than carbohydrates, the body has to work harder (uses more inhaled oxygen) to prepare the same amount of fat for energy as an equal quantity of carbohydrate.

Carbohydrates are the body's high intensity fuel. As the intensity of activity increases (muscles working harder and requiring more oxygen) the body shifts from fats to carbohydrates for energy. Although providing less than half the energy per gram as fats, carbohydrates require less oxygen to be broken down and thus are ideally suited as a high intensity fuel.

Protein has not been mentioned as an energy source, because the body will not normally utilize substantial quantities of protein as a source of energy unless the individual is severely restricted in his intake of food. Protein's primary function is the repairing and building of body tissue. Since muscle is partially composed of protein, many individuals have wrongly equated the work that muscles perform with the need to burn (use) protein for energy.


## APPLICATIONS FOR TRAINING

Recently considerable attention has been focused on the role of nutrition in athletics. Unfortunately, the scientific basis behind many nutritional practices has frequently been lacking. One point should be stressed. **No evidence exists** to prove that greatly altering a nutritionally sound diet can substantially improve the performance of an athlete. A more in-depth treatment of the role of nutrition and athletics will be presented in Chapter 10. The following considerations are discussed in terms of practical applications between nutrition and conditioning.


## CARBOHYDRATE LOADING

As previously mentioned, the body shifts to carbohydrates for energy during high intensity activity. As a result, in many instances an abundance of stored carbohydrates in the body can increase the length of time that an individual can engage in a relatively high intensity cardiovascular endurance activity, such as a marathon race. If additional carbohydrate stores within the body can improve performance in such events, a primary task facing the athlete is to increase his body's stores of this essential energy source. How can this be accomplished?

Specific techniques have been found to be effective in boosting the amount of carbohydrate stored in skeletal muscle. Generally, the process involves several steps. First, the body's carbohydrate stores must be exhausted through rigorous physical training. This should be initiated between 7 and 10 days before actual competition. Following the exhaustive training, the athlete continues to train for the next 3-4 days, but his intake of carbohydrates should be greatly reduced. For a 160lb. athlete, his daily caloric intake might consist of approximately 1500 K cal. of protein and 1300 K cal. fat. Then for 2-3 days immediately preceding competition the athlete should decrease the intensity of his workout and increase his carbohydrate intake. For the aforementioned athlete, his diet might then consist of 2300 K cal. of carboyhydrate and 500 K cal. protein. The decrease in work-out intensity with a corresponding dietary increase in carbohydrates combines to maximize glycogen (a form of carbohydrate) storage in the muscle tissues. Numerous studies investigating the performance of distance runners who used different diets have shown that the aforementioned techniques of "carbohydrate loading" generally improve the ability of the athlete to maintain a faster pace for a longer period of time.

A few words of caution, however, should be remembered concerning carbohydrate loading. Carbohydrate loading will not allow a runner to sprint faster, but it may enable him to maintain a faster pace over a greater portion of an endurance event. Secondly, carbohydrate loading should **not** be used on a weekly basis. A sound diet should be followed throughout the season, reserving the aforementioned techniques for one or two contests, **particularly long distance running events**. Additionally, the extra storage of glycogen only occurs in the muscle groups involved in the strenuous training. In other words, specificity must be judiciously followed in training so that the muscle groups involved in the sport receive the increased glycogen stores.


ROLE OF OXYGEN IN ENERGY PRODUCTION AND WORK

The break down of fats and carbohydrates supply the energy to drive the human machine. Oxygen is the primary ingredient in the scheme of energy production. With sufficient quantities of oxygen, complex chemical reactions within the body proceed to completion thereby producing the necessary energy for work. The energy material produced is in the form of a compound, known as adenosine triphosphate or ATP. When ATP, in turn, is broken down, energy is liberated to power muscular contraction. When sufficient oxygen is available for energy production, the process is known as **aerobic metabolism**. When energy is produced in the absence of an adequate supply of oxygen, it is referred to as **anaerobic metabolism**.

The level of intensity and the duration of an activity determine how ATP is produced. The body utilizes three distinct systems to produce ATP (Figure 2-1). A basic understanding of these intercellular processes of energy production will enable the athlete to develop a more effective personal training program.

## PHOSPHOGEN

The phosphogen method, known also as the ATP-PC system, is responsible for producing energy during very short, intense work bouts, normally 15 seconds or less in duration. Energy is liberated without need of oxygen and is thus one of the anaerobic systems.

The mechanism of action involved the break down of adenosine triphosphate (ATP) to adenosine diphosphate (ADP) with energy released for muscular contraction. The available supply of ATP is limited and must, somehow, be regenerated. The presence of another compound, phosocreatine (PC), assists in the regeneration of ATP. PC by itself cannot be used directly by the body for energy, but the reaction ADP + P —— ATP replenishes the ATP stores. A simplified picture of the phosphogen reactions is as follows:

(1) ATP —— ADP + inorganic P + E (used in muscular contraction)
(2) ATP —— ADP + P
Energy from (3) is used to power (2) for resynthesis of ATP.
(3) PC —— Phosphate and creatine
(4) PC —— Creatine and phosphate
Energy for (4) is derived from the aerobic metabolism of glycogen.

Athletic tasks involving primarily the phosphogen system of energy production are the 100 meter dash, the shot put, a football lineman's charge, and hitting a baseball.

The phosphogen system is a valuable means of energy production, but it has its limitations. Infinite quantities of ATP and PC do not exist in muscles. Once this system has been exhausted other methods of energy (ATP) production must take over.

## LACTIC ACID

This system derives its name from the build-up of the metabolic by-product lactic acid in the muscle and blood of the athlete. As a source of energy, the "lactic acid system" produces ATP during high intensity activities ranging from around 20 seconds up to three minutes in duration. The aerobic system assists the lactic acid system in activities lasting from 1½ to 3 minutes. ATP is initiated through the use of glucose, the end product of carbohydrate digestion. It is important to remember that because of the intensity of the exercise, carbohydrates (glucose) are the only fuel available for energy production.

Through a very complex process, the glucose molecule is split into two molecules of pyruvic acid. Although some ATP is used to accomplish the splitting, the net gain is 2 ATP molecules per molecule of glucose. If there continues to be an insufficient quantity of oxygen because of intensity of the exercise, the pyruvic acid is converted to lactic acid. When present in the blood and muscles in sufficient quantities, lactic acid acts to inhibit muscular contraction. Anyone who has ever run a 400 or 800 meter race can attest to the affect of lactic acid. The painful fatigue experienced is a direct result of it. Obviously high intensity activities, such as the aforementioned examples, can only be carried on for so long. The athlete must either cease working or lower the intensity to a level allowing for an adequate supply of oxygen to the muscles.

## AEROBIC SYSTEM

The word aerobic means with or in the presence of oxygen. The system is named after those type activities requiring large amounts of oxygen leading to development of the cardiorespiratory system. When a sufficient supply of oxygen is available to the muscles, a continuous supply of ATP is maintained. Activities utilizing primarily this system are those lasting longer than three minutes; two mile run, cross country, marathon, etc. Through this system the complete aerobic break down of one glucose molecule yields 38 molecules of ATP. Obviously it is the most efficient system the body has for energy production.

Figure 2-2 traces a molecule of glucose through the lactic acid and aerobic energy systems. The anaerobic system as depicted actually begins when in the presence of sufficient oxygen the pyruvic acid enters a complex series of reactions known as the Krebs cycle. As a result in the Krebs cycle hydrogen atoms are released and enter another series of reactions, the respiratory chain. It is here that the largest amount of ATP is produced. This is what enables an athlete to perform endurance activities for a long duration.

Figure 2-1. The energy systems of the body.

ENERGY SYSTEMS

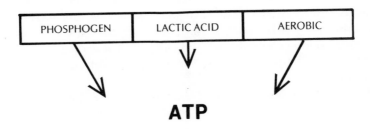

Figure 2-2. The path of a molecule of glucose through the lactic acid and aerobic energy systems.

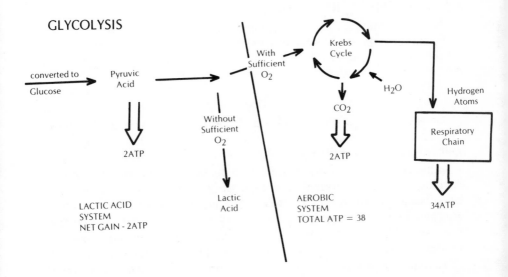

## CONTRIBUTIONS OF ENERGY SYSTEMS TO ATHLETIC PERFORMANCE

Most athletic endeavors do not derive energy from just one of the three systems, but rather a combination of two and sometimes all three. Consider the midfielder in lacrosse, the halfback in soccer, or the front row forward in rugby. Players of these positions rely heavily on the anaerobic systems because of constant short, but very intense, periods of activity during competition. They also must rely on a well developed aerobic system that will allow them to run continuously from 60-90 minutes.

The approximate contribution that each energy system makes to the athlete in the sports are listed in Figure 2-3.

## STRESS ADAPTATION

The body reacts to physical stresses upon it. The reaction may be temporary, such as the increase in an individual's heart rate during strenuous exercise; or it may be more permanent, such as the increase in the size of a muscle due to a program of strength training. This section of Chapter 2 outlines the functioning of the cardiorespiratory system and how it adapts to stress and discusses aerobic and anaerobic training considerations.

## CARDIORESPIRATORY SYSTEM

Before examining the adaptations of the heart and the lungs to exercise, the athlete should have a basic understanding of how the two systems work as a team.

## LUNGS

Air enters the mouth and nose and continues through the pharynx, larynx, and trachea into the bronchial tree. The bronchial tree has two main bronchi, one to the right lung and one to the left. The lungs may be imagined as a series of branching tubes dividing and spreading out into smaller and smaller tubules. At the end of this system lies the functional or working unit of the lungs. It is called the alveolus (plural: alveoli). The alveoli are thin sac-like structures where the exchange of oxygen and carbon dioxide take place. A thickness of one or two cells separates the air in the alveoli from the blood flowing in the capillaries.

Air enters the lungs because of pressure changes within the chest

| SPORT/ACTIVITY | PHOSPHOGEN | LACTIC ACID | AEROBIC |
|---|---|---|---|
| Baseball | 80 | 20 | |
| Basketball | 90 | 10 | |
| Field hockey | 65 | 15 | |
| Football | 95 | 15 | |
| Gymnastics | 90 | 10 | |
| Ice hockey | | | |
|   a. goalie | 100 | | |
|   b. defensemen, forwards | 70 | 30 | |
| Lacrosse | | | |
|   a. midfield | 65 | 20 | 15 |
|   b. attack, goalie, and | | | |
|     defensemen | 90 | 10 | |
| Rugby | | | |
|   a  fullback, scrum halves, | | | |
|     and backs | 90 | 10 | |
|   b. wingforwards, #8 | 60 | 20 | 20 |
|   c. front row, 2nd row | | | |
|     forwards | 40 | 40 | 20 |
| Skiing | | | |
|   a. cross country | | 10 | 90 |
|   b. downhill | 75 | 25 | |
|   c. recreational | 40 | 30 | 30 |
| Soccer | | | |
|   a. goalie, fullback, and | | | |
|     forward | 80 | 20 | |
|   b. center, halfback | 70 | 15 | 15 |
| Swimming (freestyle) | | | |
|   a. 50 meters | 95 | 5 | |
|   b. 100 meters | 75 | 15 | 10 |
|   c. 200 meters | 25 | 75 | 5 |
|   d. 400 meters | 20 | 45 | 35 |
|   e. 1500 meters | 5 | 20 | 75 |
| Track and field | | | |
|   a. 100, 200 meters | 96 | 4 | |
|   b. 400 meters | 40 | 50 | 5 |
|   c. 800 meters | 25 | 70 | 5 |
|   d. 1500 meters | 25 | 50 | 25 |
|   e. 3000 meters | 15 | 40 | 45 |
|   f. 5000 meters | 10 | 15 | 75 |
|   g. marathon | | 2 | 98 |
| Wrestling | 85 | 15 | |

Figure 2-3. The involvement of energy systems in selected sports.

cavity. As the diaphragm muscle contracts, the chest cavity is enlarged. A drop in pressure occurs lowering the air pressure in the chest cavity to a point below the outside air pressure. Air then follows the pressure gradient and rushes into the lungs. During forced inhalation, the external intercostals, scaleni, and sternocleidomastoid muscles assist the diaphragm in increasing chest cavity volume. Expiration is accomplished by the relaxation of the above muscles. The decreased chest cavity volume and increased pressure force air out of the lungs. Figure 2-4 illustrates the exchange of gases in the lung and at the tissue level.

## HEART

The human heart is divided into two halves, right and left. Each half has two chambers. Deoxygenated venous blood coming back to the heart from the body enters the right atrium. From there it goes into the right ventricle. Here it is pumped out of the heart to the lungs. In the lungs, oxygen is picked up and carbon dioxide ($CO_2$) deposited for expiration. The single cell thickness between the blood capillaries and alveoli facilitates this exchange. The $CO_2$ leaves the body during normal lung expiration. This gas exchange comes about because of pressure differences. Obviously the pressure of $O_2$ in the alveoli is greater than in the venous blood coming into the lungs. The reverse is true for carbon dioxide. Gases move from areas of high pressure to low pressue. Thus the exchange takes place. At the tissue level, the exchange is reversed. The oxygenated blood then leaves the lungs, returning to the left atrium. It then goes to the left ventricle and is pumped out of the heart to the body. Once at the cell level, $O_2$ is transferred into the cell for work and the cells' waste products, to include $CO_2$, move into the blood capillary. Through the venous system the blood is delivered again to the right atrium. Figure 2-5 illustrates the blood flow through the heart.

ADAPTIONS TO EXERCISE

In order to better understand how the body reacts to exercise, a few points of how the body functions during **normal, non-strenuous activity** should be examined. The heart rate for an average male is around 72 beats per minute. A normal heart ejects around 5000 milliliters of blood to the body per minute. At the tissue level approximately 25% of the available oxygen typically is transferred from the blood into the cells.

During strenuous exercise, things are much different. Breathing becomes markedly heavier. The intercostals, scaleni, and sternocleidomastoid assist the diaphragm in varying the volume of the chest cavity.

Figure 2-4. The exchange of gases in the lung and at the tissue level.

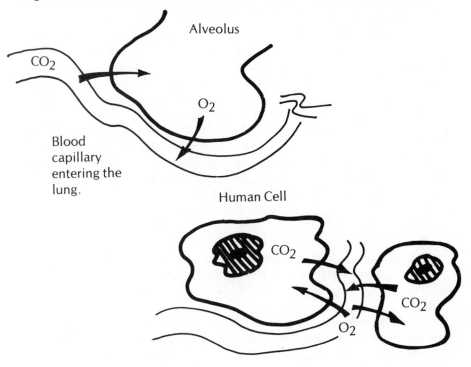

Figure 2-5. Blood flow through the heart.

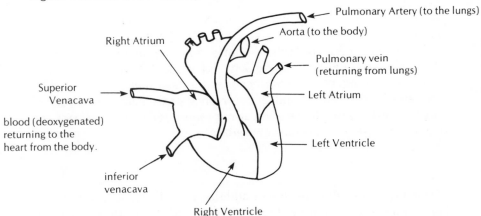

The heart rate increases, and if the exercise is strenuous enough, it may go as high as 180-200 beats per minute. The amount of blood pumped per beat also increases. Due to stimulation by the nervous system, the heart muscle contracts harder forcing out more blood with each beat. This is known as stroke volume. If the stroke volume and heart rate both increase, the total blood pumped per minute (cardiac output) also increases. In fact, from an average resting level of 5000 ml. a minute, cardiac output may reach 25,000 ml. per minute during heavy exercise. It may go as high as 38,000 ml. in a trained athlete.

Adaptations take place also at the tissue level. During heavy exercise approximately 75-80% of the oxygen in the capillaries is transferred to the cells. With five times the cardiac output and a threefold increase in oxygen deliverance, the total oxygen available to the muscle is approximately 15 times the resting level, a substantial difference.

## LONG TERM ADAPTATIONS

The following adaptations resulting from conditioning occur in the cardio-respiratory system over a prolonged period of time.

### Heart

Since the heart is composed of muscle, it responds to heavy work in the same manner as does skeletal muscle. It enlarges in size. The walls between chambers thicken enabling more forceful contractions. The stronger the contractions, the greater the stroke volume. Thus resting heart rate lowers without any loss in cardiac output. These factors combine to make the heart a more efficient pump.

### Lungs

Continual overloading of the respiratory muscles increases their level of strength, endurance, and capacity for work. Interior lung volume increases creating a greater surface area for gas exchange. As a result, more alveoli are utilized and the efficiency of exchange is improved. This all translates into lowered breathing rates during periods of rest and smaller increases during bouts of exercise.

### Capillaries

Training causes the opening of additional capillary beds in both the lungs and the musculature. Obviously the entire exchange process is improved.

## Blood

Well conditioned athletes have greater blood volumes than their unconditioned counterparts. Greater blood volume increases the circulatory system's ability to transport nutrients to the muscles. Blood content also changes with training. Trained individuals have a larger percentage of red blood cells per unit of whole blood. Oxygen is carried on a portion of the red blood cell, the hemaglobin molecule, and with more red cells, its carrying capacity is increased.

## Muscle Glycogen Stores

Conditioning increases the amount of muscle glycogen stored in the muscles involved in the training. This increases the athlete's capacity for endurance work. Depending on the type of training, increased ATP and PC stores may also be present.

## AEROBIC TRAINING

In order to increase the aerobic capacity of an athlete, a demand must be placed on his cardiovascular system. How is this accomplished? In general, the individual is required to work out on a regular basis (3 or 4 times a week) at a relatively high level of intensity (approximately 70-80% of his maximum heart rate for most individuals, 140-150 beats per minute), and for an extended period of time (at least 15-20 minutes per workout). Specific programs for aerobic development are presented in Chapter 13.

## ANAEROBIC TRAINING

As was mentioned earlier, in the absence of oxygen, anaerobic processes supply ATP for muscular contraction. Oxygen is not available because the work intensity is too great to allow aerobic production of ATP. These anaerobic processes are very important in events requiring maximum effort for short intervals. the 200 and 400 meter sprints are classic examples of anaerobic eents. The short bursts of speed required in nearly all team sports are also accomplished with anaerobic reserves.

Anaerobic fitness is developed through short intense work bouts. Fast interval training is ideally suited for this (see Chapter 13). Caution must be exercised in structuring the work bout duration. It should be as close as possible to the time of the actual competition. The athlete who wants to lower his quarter mile run time should engage in anaerobic work bouts, each about one minute in duration. Running a series of 15-

second, 100 meter sprints would not accomplish the desired goal. Current research points to one minute as the minimum work interval time for maximizing anaerobic endurance, particularly for the Lactic Acid system.

Individuals who want to develop the most effective training program possible should include training activities in their programs which involve energy sources in approximations similar to their specific sport (see Figure 2-3).

Figure 2-6 lists the energy systems involved in ten of the most popular forms of training.

| TYPE OF TRAINING | PHOSPHOGEN | LACTIC ACID | AEROBIC |
| --- | --- | --- | --- |
| Acceleration sprinting | 90 | 5 | 5 |
| Repetition sprints | 90 | 6 | 4 |
| Jog sprints | 85 | 10 | 5 |
| Fast interval | 30 | 50 | 20 |
| Fartlek training | 20 | 40 | 40 |
| Interval sprints | 20 | 10 | 70 |
| Repetition running | 10 | 50 | 40 |
| Slow interval | 10 | 30 | 60 |
| Continuous fast running | — | 10 | 90 |
| Long slow distance running | — | 5 | 95 |

Figure 2-6. The percentage of contribution of the energy systems to selected types of training.

KEY:

**Acceleration sprinting:** gradual increase in speed from jogging to sprinting. One might jog 25 meters, run ½-¾ speed for 25 meters, then sprint for 50 meters.

**Repetition running:** involves distances generally from one-half to three miles with complete recovery (walking) in between.

**Interval running:** involves running with only incomplete recovery (jogging) between work bouts. Work bouts are submaximal in intensity. See below for explanation of types of intervals.

**Fast interval:** well suited for pre-season regime where specificity and anaerobic power are paramount. Intensity of the work interval is greater than in slow interval (¾ speed). Athlete should jog during the relief interval. Heart rate should reach 180 BPM after successive intervals.

**Slow interval:** formal fast-slow running. The work interval is accomplished at roughly ½-¾ speed, and the heart rate should reach 180 BPM after successive work bouts. Jogging is done during the relief interval and normally is three times the duration of the work interval. Intensity of the work interval is greater than in continuous fast running.

**Jog-sprints:** sprinting followed by equal distance of jogging between the sprints.

**Fartlek:** informal slow-fast running over varied terrain. It combines all forms of training.

**Interval sprints:** short sprints (50-60 meters) followed by jogging (20-30 meters followed again by sprints for two- three miles total distance).

**Repetition sprints:** maximum performance over short distances with near complete recovery (pulse dropping below 120BPM).

**Long slow-distance running:** running long distances at slow pace (jogging). Heart rate should be around 140-150 BPM.

**Continuous fast running:** pace is faster than in slow running. It is designed to allow the body to adapt to increasing work loads.

# CHAPTER 3
## Strength Training: Fundamentals and Techniques

Daniel P. Riley
Director of Strength Training

Warm-up
Muscle size and strength
Muscle soreness
Proper training techniques
Spotters
Breathing
Safety considerations
Rubber sweat suits
Exercise antagonists
Exercise thru the full range of movement
Positive versus negative work
Emphasize negative work
Intensity
Grips
Record workout data

The first requirement for an effective weight training program is the learning of the basic skills and guidelines attendant to a properly conducted strength development program. Adherence to these fundamental precepts will enable athletes to accomplish two objectives: (1) train in as safe a manner as is possible; and (2) maximize their gains in muscular development.

WARM-UP
Although contradictory information exists regarding the possible benefits of warming- or limbering-up before training with weights, common sense dictates that some energy should be devoted to a warm-up period if for no other than safety reasons. Since warming-up produces an increase in the internal temperature of the body which in turn affects the elasticity and extensibility of the involved muscle tissue, the individual who "warms-up" before engaging in rigorous activity is generally believed to be less prone to muscle pulls, tears, etc. The length of the warm-up period and the activities to be followed depend on the individual. For most individuals, five to ten minutes of limbering-up should suffice. Suggested warm-up activities include: jumping-jacks, running-in-place, and lifting **light** weights through the ranges of motion specific to the exercise in the weight training program.

## MUSCLE SIZE AND STRENGTH

When a demand is placed on a muscle, the muscle responds to the stress by growing in size, also referred to hypertrophying. This growth is the result of an increase in the size (**not the number**) of the individual fibers and the tissue (fascia) which surrounds the fibers. The strength of a muscle is roughly proportional to its cross-sectional area. All other factors being equal, the larger the muscle, the stronger the muscle.

## MUSCLE SORENESS

In the initial stages of a properly conducted weight training program, an individual exerts tension on infrequently used or unused muscle fibers. This tension causes waste products (specifically lactic acid and carbon dioxide) to accumulate faster than the body can use or remove them. These waste products are believed to bring about the feeling of soreness by sensitizing local pain receptors. The best method for relieving muscle soreness and stiffness is to train for three or four successive days at a level of normal workout intensity. After this initial conditioning stage, all muscle soreness should disappear. Any subsequent introduction of new movements in the training program will result in some soreness. Temporary relief of muscle soreness can be achieved by applying heat and massage to the affected muscles in order to speed up circulation, thereby abetting the removal of the aforementioned waste products.

## PROPER TRAINING TECHNIQUES

A complete mastery of the basic techniques of weight training is a critical factor in the degree of success the athlete can achieve in strength training program. Without total adherence to the correct techniques, the exercises cannot be performed properly; the individual cannot capitalize on his existing potential for improvement; and the trainee's susceptibility to injury is increased. All athletes should become **totally familiar** with the basic techniques for performing each exercise which are described in detail in Chapters 5 and 6. The individual who is lifting weights for the first time should devote the first one or two workouts to practicing the basic movements involved in each exercise with relatively light resistance in order to gain a working familiarity of the proper techniques.

## SPOTTERS

Spotters are individuals who assist someone engaged in lifting weights. This assistance may be before, during, or after the completion of an exercise. A spotter has two primary responsibilities: (1) Prevent injuries to either the lifter or anyone in the adjacent vicinity, and (2) provide assistance to the lifter which facilitates the proper execution of the exercise (e.g. bring a heavy weight into the starting position for an exercise).

A spotter can also aid the lifter by providing constant verbal feedback. Such feedback can stimulate the desire of the lifter to achieve an "all-out effort" by discouraging him from quitting when the discomfort becomes stressful. Verbal encouragement also helps reinforce proper training techniques. Frequently, as the lifter becomes more fatigued, his adherence to correct form gradually decreases unless told to perform otherwise. In negative-only training (see the section of this Chapter on "EMPHASIZE NEGATIVE WORK") the spotter often assumes additional major responsibilities.

The guidelines for serving as a spotter are basic. During most exercises, come from beneath the weight (not over it) in order to prevent the weight from falling on the lifter. Remember that the last repetition, if performed properly, has a substantial effect on the degree of improvement achievement by the lifter. Allow the lifter to do as much work as possible on his final repetition. A final note — **NO ONE** should assume the responsibilities of a spotter unless he is aware of the proper spotting techniques.


BREATHING

Breathing while engaged in weight training should be synchronized with the exercise. There is a physiological need for breathing during each and every repetition of any exercise. Adherence to the proper breathing pattern facilitates the function and efficiency of an exercise. The most consistent and efficient method that can be utilized in determining how to breathe properly is to inhale whenever the resistance is being lowered or pulled toward the body and exhale when the resistance moves away from the body (e.g. blow the weight away from the body).

The lifter should never hold his breath while training. On occasion, an inexperienced lifter holds his breath in order to "gut out" an extra repetition. More-often-than-not, this practice results in a decrease in the efficiency of the exercise. In addition, holding one's breath while training can also produce either dizziness or unconsciousness. This condition is the result of the Valsalva Phenomenon. This phenomenon results from the buildup of inner thoracic (inner rib cage) pressure due to the great pressure or force of a weight on an individual's body who is holding his breath. This pressure, built up inside the rib cage, compresses the right side of the heart which in turn restricts the flow of blood, and consequently $O_2$ to the entire body. Some exercises bring on the symptoms of the Valsalva Phenomenon more readily than others (i.e. squat, seated or military press, deadlift, biceps curl, bench press).

## SAFETY CONSIDERATIONS

For the individual who adheres to proper lifting techniques and utilizes a reasonable level of common sense, weight lifting is a relatively safe activity. Most injuries result from either carelessness or ignorance. The following guidelines should be followed:

- Never train with weights at a high level of intensity without having mastered the techniques involved in performing the exercise.
- Use spotters whenever necessary.
- Always make sure that plate collars for the free weights are securely tightened.
- Wear footwear in order to cushion the blow from a falling object and to avoid stubbing the toes.
- When loading or unloading one side of a barbell, load or unload the other side evenly.
- Remember that the weight room is not a playroom. Be considerate of others.

## RUBBER SWEAT SUITS

Perspiring is the body's mechanism for preventing overheating. When the temperature of the body rises, the perspiration process begins. Evaporation of perspiration cools the body surface which in turn helps control body temperature. Covering the body with a plastic or rubber sweat suit prevents the natural cooling down process of the body to take place. The heat produced is not dissipated, and the temperature of the body continues to rise. This causes a rise in blood pressure and overtaxes the heart. Simply stated, these suits serve no practical purpose in a strength training program (or any other properly conducted conditioning program for that matter).

## EXERCISE ANTAGONISTS

Pairs of muscle groups which oppose each other are called antagonists (e.g. the biceps and the triceps). Practically every muscle in the body has an antagonist. To develop one muscle or group of muscles upsets the equilibrium of the opposing muscles. As a muscle becomes stronger than its antagonist, the flexibility of the joint controlled by the

31

affected musculature is decreased. As a result, both the joint and the involved muscles are more susceptible to injury.

Many athletes are frequently guilty of not achieving a balance of strength in opposing muscle groups. Such individuals can be seen exercising the quadriceps by running hills, stadium steps, riding bicycles, etc., but ignoring the hamstrings. This leads to a loss in flexibility and strength in the hamstrings in relation to the quadriceps and leaves the hamstrings more susceptible to pulls and tears.

Another muscle group often over-developed are the pectorals (chest muscles). If a lifter exercises only the chest muscles, and not the antagonist (upper back muscles), the pectorals become stronger than the muscles of the upper back. The muscles of the chest then gradually pull the shoulder girdle forward which may cause a condition known as "round shouldered" (Figure 3-1). As a result, when developing a weight training program, the athlete should always include an exercise for the antagonist of all exercises included in the program.

## EXERCISE THROUGH A FULL RANGE OF MOVEMENT

Flexibility, one of the primary components of physical fitness, is defined as the capacity of a joint to move through a full range of movement. The primary factor affecting that capacity is the musculature surrounding the joint. When the joint is periodically required to go through a full range of motion, the involved muscles retain their natural elasticity. When a joint is not utilized through its full range of movement on a regular basis, the surrounding musculature tends to tighten-up, causing it to lose some of its elasticity. As a result, the joint becomes less flexible. For the athlete, the loss of flexibility can result in a decrease in his ability to perform and increase the chances for injury.

Contrary to superstition and unfounded myths, properly performed weight training exercises actually increase flexibility. In fact, it is impossible for an athlete who exercises through a **full range of movement** to decrease his flexibility. Adherence to correct lifting techniques will enable the athlete to develop strength throughout the entire range of movement for his body's musculature.

## POSITIVE VERSUS NEGATIVE WORK

Two distinctive movements can be observed when an individual is performing a weight training exercise: The raising of the weight and the lowering of the weight. The raising of the weight is considered **positive work** and the lowering of the weight **negative work.** When performing positive work the muscle is shortening (contracting). While lowering the

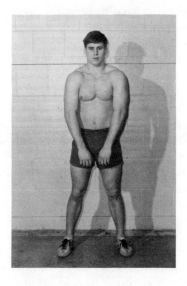

Figure 3-1. An example of a
round shouldered condition.

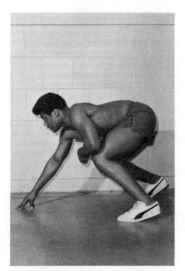

Figure 3-2.
Football player's stance.

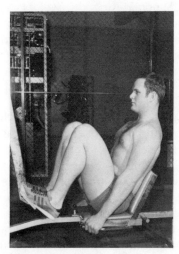

Figure 3-3. Leg press.

Figures 3-2 and 3-3 illustrate the close relationship between the
flexibility required for a specific sport's task (football player's stance)
and the range of motion involved in the proper execution of a specific
weight training exercise (leg press).

weight the muscle is lengthened. The muscles used to raise the weight are the same muscles used to lower the weight.

For example, when lifting the weight while performing the biceps curl, the muscle is performing work while it is shortening. When the weight is lowered, the same muscle group is performing the work. In this instance, however, the biceps are lengthening.

The negative portion of an exercise is just as important as the positive movement. Unfortunately, negative work is often ignored by individuals engaged in weight training. Since it is easier to lower than it is to raise that same weight, the tendency is to be less conscious of form when lowering the weight. Both movements however should be performed as exacting as possible, perhaps placing even a greater emphasis on the lowering of the weight. It should take a longer period of time to lower the weight than it did to raise it.

Many athletes "throw" a weight rather than allow the muscles to lift it. They generate enough momentum so that the exercise becomes a ballistic movement. The body will recruit fewer fibers to perform this kind of exercise. "Throwing" the weight can be observed in many exercises but it is particularly obvious in an exercise such as the leg extension.

When raising the weight, the athlete should control the weight's speed of movement. The lifter should be able to stop the weight at any time during the "positive" movement. The weight should not be bounced or jerked during any part of the range of movement for an exercise.


EMPHASIS ON NEGATIVE WORK TRAINING

In the previous section it was stated that the negative portion of the exercise is as important (and some researchers believe it is more important) as the positive part of the exercise. When performing an exercise to the point of momentary muscular failure, the individual will eventually fail during the positive portion of the exercise. That is to say, he is no longer capable of "raising" the weight through the full range of movement. When he has reached this point, he has generally obtained maximum benefit from this portion of the program. A muscle, however, is capable of lowering much more weight than it can raise. Even though the muscle has failed during the positive portion of the exercise, it could continue to perform additional **negative work**. The point of momentary muscular failure for the negative portion of the exercise is much greater than for the positive movement. Therefore, the lifter has not maximized his potential for gain from an exercise when he quits at the point when he no longer can lift a weight through the positive phase. The only way to obtain the maximum benefits from the negative portion of the exercise is to periodically take the muscles to the point of momentary muscular failure during the negative portion of the exercise. To accomplish this, the lifter must perform some type of training that places an emphasis on the negative part of the exercise.

There are two techniques that can be utilized to perform this function. These techniques are **negative only** training and **negative accentuated** training.

When performing **negative only exercise**, the individual only engages in the negative portion of the exercise. In short, he only lowers the weight. To perform negative only exercise, the lifter needs either spotters to raise the weight for him or equipment that is specifically designed for negative only training.

The following guidelines for performing **negative only training** are recommended:

The athlete should use as much resistance as possible so that:

1. At any point during repetitions 1-4, he can stop the descent of the resistance and momentarily change direction.

2. At any point during repetitions 5-8, he can stop the descent of the resistance and pause momentarily but are unable to change direction.

3. During repetitions 9 and 10, he is unable to momentarily stop the descent of the resistance.

Figures 3-4, 3-5, and 3-6 illustrate a technique that may be used when performing negative only chinups.

Negative only exercise can be of great value to the athlete who is lacking the requisite muscular development to properly perform a particular exercise. For example, if he can only perform 2 pullups, it will take him a great deal of time before he is capable of performing 2¼, 2½, 3, 3¼ etc. In general, two or three complete repetitions of any exercise is not enough to stimulate maximum gains in muscular development. In this instance, however, he could continue to improve by performing negative only pullups. By continuing to lower his body weight after he is no longer capable of performing the positive portion of the pullup, he will be strengthening the same muscles used to raise his body weight.

It is very difficult to perform some exercises in the negative only fashion, since either specially designed equipment or several spotters would be needed to raise the weight for the lifter. Another technique which can be used to emphasize the negative part of the exercise is the "**negative accentuated**" method of excercising.

During negative accentuated exercise, the individual lifts the weight with two appendages and lowers it with one. Obviously, it is very difficult to perform **negative accentuated exercise** without the use of

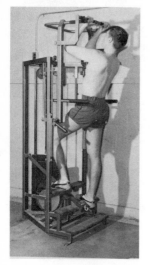

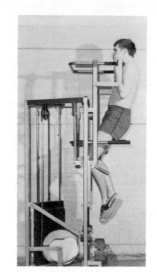

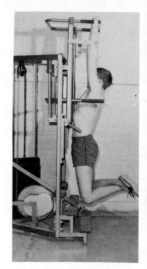

| Figure 3-4* | Figure 3-5* | Figure 3-6* |

*Techniques for performing **negative-only** chinups.

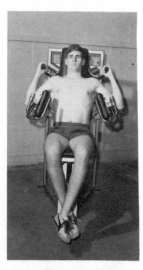

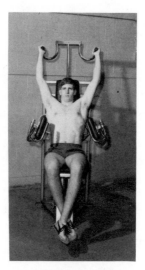

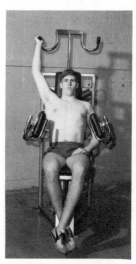

| Figure 3-7** | Figure 3-8** | Figure 3-9** |

**Techniques for performing a **negative-accentuated** exercise.

either a Nautilus or a Universal machine.

Figure 3-7, 3-8, and 3-9 illustrate an individual exercising in the negative accentuated fashion using a Nautilus machine. If, for example, an individual could perform this exercise in normal fashion at a level of 10 repetitions with 100 pounds, he would be able to substantially increase the resistance a single limb would be required to overcome by exercising in a negative accentuated fashion. That is to say, he would raise the weight with two hands and lower it with one. In this instance, on his first repetition, he would lower 100 pounds with his right hand and then would alternate and lower the weight on the next repetition with his left hand. By definition, negative accentuated exercise "accentuates" the negative portion of the exercise. This type of training allows the athlete to approach the point of momentary muscular failure during the negative portion of the exercise. Momentary muscular failure during the raising of the weight while performing negative accentuated exercise will still be experienced however.

The following guidelines for performing negative accentuated exercises are recommended:

1. Use as much weight as possible so that you fail somewhere between 8-12 repetitions. One repetition constitutes the raising of the weight in both arms or legs then lowering it in one arm or leg.

2. Eliminate all bouncing or jerking movements when making the transfer of weight from two appendages to one.

3. The non-working arm or leg should be ready to immediately initiate the raising of the weight as soon as the resistance has been completely lowered.

As can be observed from Figure 3-10, there are advantages of performing all three methods of training (normal, negative only, negative accentuated).

| | Normal | Negative Only | Negative Accentuated |
|---|---|---|---|
| Intensity during the positive portion of the exercise | Maximum | Non-Existent | Maximum |
| Intensity during the negative portion of the exercise | Moderate | Maximum | Moderately High |

Figure 3-10.

# Strength Training: Fundamentals and Techniques

In order to obtain the best of what each type of training has to offer and to minimize tedium in the training, it is strongly recommended that the methods of training employed in the conditioning program be varied periodically.

## INTENSITY

The higher the level of intensity exhibited by the athlete in a weight training program the greater his increase in muscle development. The level of intensity is determined by three factors: (1) the effort extended by the individual; (2) the use of proper training methods and techniques; and (3) the equipment used in the conditioning program.

The effort that is extended is the most important of these three elements. The greater the effort extended, the higher the intensity of the exercise. The effort being extended reaches its maximum when the lifter reaches the point of momentary muscle failure. That is, the individual trains to the point where the muscle being exercised has failed momentarily and can no longer execute another properly performed repetition. For example, while performing the squatting exercise the lifter will eventually reach a point when he can no longer recover from the squatting position to the starting position (standing). A 100% effort has not been extended by the lifter if he does not reach the point of momentary muscular failure.

Equipment that varies the resistance is essential for **maximum** muscle fiber recruitment throughout the entire range of movement, such equipment varies the resistance to accomodate the various strength curves of the body, thereby producing a greater recruitment of muscle fibers. Regardless of the equipment being used, a maximum effort must be extended and all the proper training techniques must be observed to achieve high level intensity and maximum gains in muscular development.

The athlete who is interested in training at a level of high intensity should make an attempt to experience high intensity exercise in order to evaluate his present conditioning program. In most instances, athletes simply are unaware of what constitutes a high intensity effort. Frankly, it is almost impossible when training alone to reach the point of momentary muscular failure. The use of a training partner is the most effective tool for the athlete who wants to push himself to his physical (and sometimes psychological) limits.

The athlete should remember that there is a minimum level of intensity at which he can train and still continue to improve his level of muscular development. Although he can train at a point past the minimum required level and achieve gains, the athlete should keep in mind that a less-than-maximum effort will produce less-than-maximum results.


## GRIPS

There are four grips that can be used when performing the various barbell exercises. These grips are the overhand, the underhand, the alternate, and the false grip.

1. The **overhand grip** is the most widely used grip when performing the barbell exercises. The thumbs are hooked underneath the bar with the knuckles placed on top of the bar. (Figure 3-11).

2. When the **underhand grip** is used, the thumbs are hooked above the bar and the knuckles are placed underneath the bar (Fig. 3-12).

3. When using the **alternate grip**, a combination of the overhand and the underhand grip is used. One hand is placed above and one hand below the bar (Fig. 3-13). The alternate grip is the strongest grip of the four. It can be used when performing an exercise similar to the deadlift or shoulder shrug.

4. When using the **false grip** the thumbs are not hooked around the bar. It is a grip that should not be used by a novice lifter. It can be a substitute for the overhand or underhand grip when performing certain exercises. It is often susbtituted because it is a more comfortable grip. However, as it's name implies it is not a very safe grip (Fig. 3-14).

The width of the particular grip being used varies with the individual and the exercise being performed. The width of the grip should provide the following: (1) maximum range of movement; (2) isolation of the specific muscle or group of muscles being exercised; and (3) comfort.

The grip should be consistent when performing the same exercise. For example, each and every time the lifter performs the bench press, he should use the same width grip.


## RECORD WORKOUT DATA

During each workout, the amount of resistance lifted and the number of repetitions performed for **each** exercise should be recorded. This recording helps eliminate the duplication of a previous workout and provides incentive for improvement. Since during a single workout an athlete frequently performs many exercises, and repetitions with varying workloads, it is generally quite difficult to recall from one workout to another the specific accomplishments of prior training sessions. As a result, unless a record is kept of all workout data, the danger exists that an individual will not make the regular program adjustments which are necessary for self-improvement. Figure 3-15 provides an example

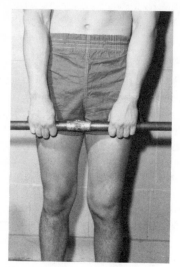

Figure 3-11. Overhand grip.

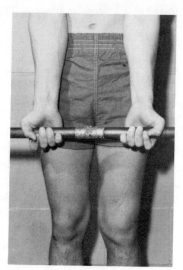

Figure 3-12. Underhand grip

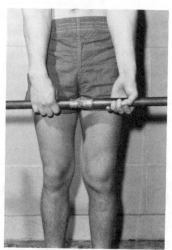

Figure 3-13. Alternate grip.

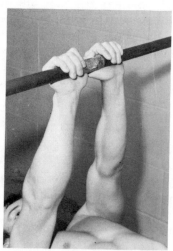

Figure 3-14. False grip.

Figure 3-15. A sample workout card.

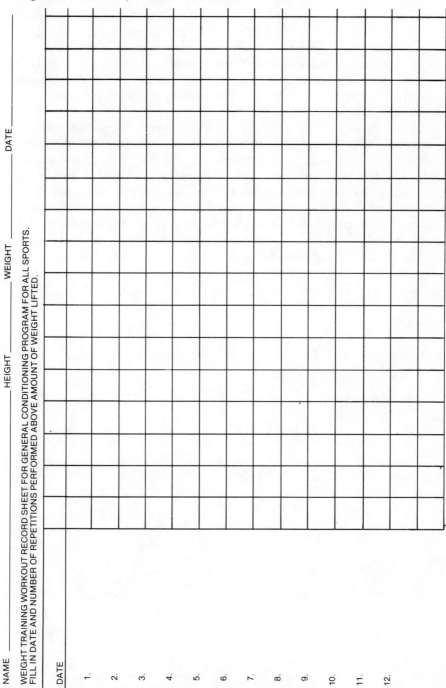

of of a typical workout card. Note that the date of the training session, the exercise in the program, the amount of resistance for each exercise, and the number of repetitions each exercise was performed are recorded.

Recording workout data also provides the athlete with an **incentive** for increasing the amount of resistance or the number of repetitions he can perform on each exercise. If for example, an athlete performed 8 repetitions using 100 pounds of a particular exercise on his last workout, his goal should now be to try and and perform at least 9 repetitions with that same weight.

A record of workout data can also serve as a **measuring stick for improvement.** As such, it can serve as an invaluable tool for the coach who wants to monitor the performance of his athletes. As a general rule, the athlete should strive for a certain degree of continual progress in muscular development. The gradual improvement in performance in the weight training room often serves as a stimulant for maintaining a personal commitment to the conditioning program. Eventually, the athlete will receive more substantial feedback from his conditioning efforts in the form of improved performance in the athletic area.

# CHAPTER 4
## Organizing a Strength Training Program

Daniel P. Riley
Director of Strength Training

Program prerequisites
Program objectives
Seven training variables

A muscular development program should be organized to meet three basic criteria: **soundness, functionability,** and **efficiency.** A program is **sound** when it is based on scientific principles and research. Unfortunately, the body of knowledge related to weight lifting is replete with innuendos, superstitions, and unfounded half-truths. Too often, the novice lifter is forced to rely on the empirical practices and ideas of friends and athletic coaches. The vast majority of printed matter on the subject is also limited—both in scope and in reliabilty. For the athlete, the main task is to separate **fact** from **fiction** and then develop a program based on scientifically-proven fact.

A program is **functional** if it is specific in developing the muscular develoment required to meet the objectives of the athlete's conditioning program. For example, if one of the athlete's goals is to improve their jumping ability, they should include exercises specific to the musculature involved in jumping (e.g. leg press and leg extension).

A program is **efficient** if it produces muscular development in the athlete as rapidly as possible, subject to the individual's capacity (potential) for improvement. In evaluating a program's efficiency, the following question must be asked: "Could the athlete have achieved the same results (and in some instances, possibly better results) from a program which utilized different training techniques and required either **less** training time or **less** work output by the lifter?" If the answer to this question is "yes", then the program is not as efficient as it could be.

PROGRAM PREREQUISITES

In order to organize an effective muscular development program, the athlete should become familiar with the following: (1) the muscles and muscle groups of the body; (2) the function (action) of each muscle during physical activity; and (3) a specific exercise to develop each involved muscle or muscle group. Figures 4-1 and 4-2 illustrate the primary muscles of the body. An overview of the role of each muscle in athletics is presented in Chapter 13.

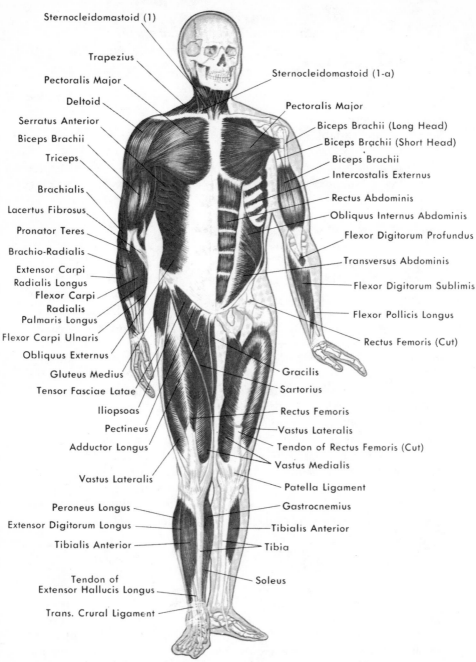

Figure 4-1. Muscles of the body: anterior view (Reprinted by permission of Cramer Products Inc.)

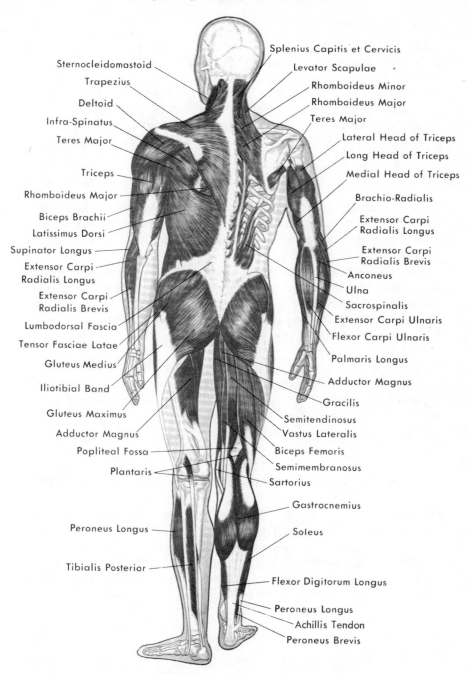

Figure 4-2. Muscles of the body: posterior view. (Reprinted by permission of Cramer Products Inc.)

## PROGRAM OBJECTIVES

One of the first steps in organizing a muscular development program is to establish program objectives. Although there are a wide variety of secondary reasons for participating in a lifting program—vanity, personal fitness, sports ability improvement, etc.—all are predicated upon the individual raising his/her level of muscular development. Muscular development programs can be grouped into four general categories: bodybuilding, rehabilitation, competitive lifting, and weight training.

## BODYBUILDING

**Bodybuilding** is the term used to collectively categorize the goals of individuals who lift to improve the appearance of their bodies. There is a large spectrum of bodybuilders ranging from 90 pound weaklings to Mr. Americas. Within this large spectrum of bodybuilders are those individuals who possess different levels of interest for developing the body. The most advanced level of bodybuilding is competitive bodybuilding. Primarily a male domain, the competitive bodybuilder develops his body to prepare for competition where the "best developed" man is declared the victor. In such competition, the judges evaluate body symmetry, muscle mass and definition, and posing ability. Another popular reason for bodybuilding is to change body weight. Individuals who want to gain weight try to develop additional muscle mass; while individuals who want to lose weight, attempt to firm up by increasing their level of muscle tonus.

## REHABILITATION

Strength training plays an important role in rehabilitating the athlete to pre-injury levels of fitness and in minimizing the possibility of re-injury. Injured athletes should proceed judiciously in organizing their "redevelopment" programs. Guidance from either a physician or a certified trainer should be obtained and followed. Strength training also can play a role in **preventing** injuries. Well-developed and toned muscles, in concert with adequate levels of flexibility, decreases the potential of muscle pulls and strains, as well as, ligament trauma.

## COMPETITIVE TRAINING

Organized competition between individuals (and sometimes teams) to see who can lift the most weight is called competitive lifting. Grouped according to bodyweight, the lifters compete against individ-

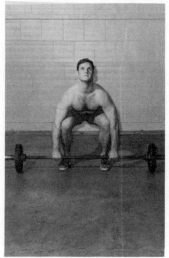

Figure 4-3*

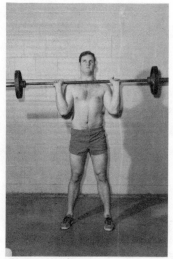

Figure 4-4*

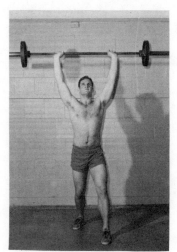

Figure 4-5*

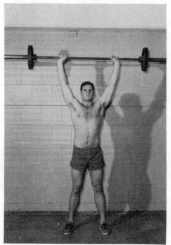

Figure 4-6*

*The "Clean and Jerk."

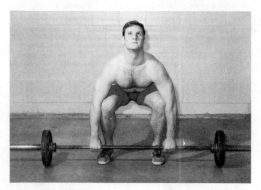

Figure 4-7*

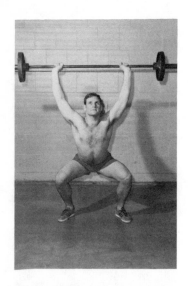

Figure 4-8*

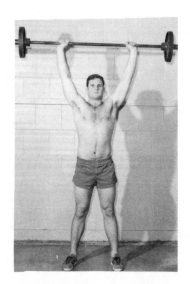

Figure 4-9*

*The "snatch."

uals of similar weight. Depending upon the level of competition, very specific rules govern all lifting.

The AAU sanctions two types of competition: Olympic lifting and power lifting. Having their origins in the Olympic games, there are two Olympic lifts—the clean and jerk (Fig. 4-3, 4-4, 4-5, and 4-6) and the snatch (Fig. 4-7, 4-8, and 4-9). In previous years, a third Olympic lift existed—military press. The military press was eliminated however, because it was a very difficult lift to judge.

Both Olympic lifts start with the barbell resting on the floor and finish with the bar in the arms extended position overhead. The Olympic lifter must combine speed, strength, explosive power, coordination, and a great deal of technique to achieve a high level of proficiency.

There are three lifts that compose the power lifts: the squat, the bench press, and the deadlift. When performing the power lifts, the bar travels a shorter distance as compared to the Olympic lifts. To achieve a high level of proficiency, the lifter must possess a high level of strength, power, and technique.

It is possible for individuals to engage in competitive lifting without taking part in an AAU sanctioned meet. They may compete with a friend in the weight room to establish who can lift the most weight on a specific exercise. They also could fulfill requirements of a test of some sort (coaches measuring strength of a team, instructor measuring progress in a strength development class, etc.).

## WEIGHT TRAINING

The primary objective of a weight training program is to improve the trainee's level of muscular development so that the lifter's ability to perform a specific physical task will also be improved. In general, most weight training programs are designed to improve athletic ability. It is no understatement that "a stronger athlete is a better athlete." All athletes should strive to substantially increase their level of muscular development during the off-season and should attempt to at least maintain their pre-season level of muscular development during the season. All too frequently, coaches and athletes discontinue their weight training programs during the season resulting in a dramatic loss of muscular development in the athletes by the end of the season.

## THE SEVEN TRAINING VARIABLES

The actual organization of an efficient strength development program involves the manipulation of seven training variables. While there may be hundreds of possibilities in which these training variables could be manipulated, the following recommendations are the most efficient methods available for improving muscular development. To deviate from the prescribed methods mentioned herein will produce "**less**" than maximum gains in muscular development. The program organization for both male and female athletes is the identical.

In this day and age of specialization, the athlete frequently devotes many hours practicing, developing, and improving the skills needed to excel in a specific sport or athletic event. Accordingly, the time spent in the weight training room should be organized as efficiently as possible. Based upon the existing literature and the most current research, proper manipulation of the following seven training variables will produce the most efficient, personalized strength training program:

1. The number of repetitions to be performed.
2. The number of sets to be performed.
3. The amount of weight to be used during each exercise (workload).
4. The time interval between exercises.
5. The frequency of workout.
6. The exercises to be performed.
7. The order of exercise.

## REPETITION

A **repetition** (rep) is the number of times a lift is executed. For maximum muscle fiber recruitment and development, between 8 and 12 repetitions of each exercise should be performed. If at least 8 repetitions of an exercise cannot be done, then the weight is too heavy. If more than 12 repetitions of an exercise can be done, then the weight is too light.

For maximum efficiency, exercise should be continued until a properly executed repetition can no longer be performed (this should happen between 8 and 12 reps). If the athlete stops short of this point of momentary muscular failure, he/she will not gain as much from that particular exercise as he/she could have. Keep in mind that a **submaximal** effort will produce **submaximal** results.

## SET

A **set** consists of the total number of repetitions executed each time an exercise is performed. When using conventional barbell equipment two sets of 8-12 repetitions are recommended. These two sets should be performed consecutively, using the proper weight lifting technique. When using equipment that varies the resistance (i.e., nautilus, universal gym, isokinetic machine) only one set should be performed. It is **how** the exercise is performed that produces results not **how much** exercise is done.

Check points for a properly performed set include the following:

1. Raise the weight using the required muscles, as opposed to throwing the weight (at least 2 seconds to raise the weight).

2. Emphasize the lowering of the weight. The same muscle that was used to raise the weight should also be used to lower the weight (at least 4 seconds to lower the weight).

3. Exert an all-out effort until eventually reaching the point of momentary muscular failure (unable to perform another properly executed repetition) somewhere between 8 and 12 repetitions.

4. Exercise through the full range of movement.

The human body is only capable of recovering from a specific amount of exercise. Exceeding this arbitrary expenditure of energy makes additional exercise counterproductive. In theory, and in practice, the fewer the number of sets which are performed, the easier it is for the body to recover from the demands of the exercise. The body cannot fully recover from multiple sets of **properly** executed exercise. Progress is actually retarded by performing additional sets.

Unfortunately, much has been written about athletes who perform many sets of an exercise and who have increased substantially their level of physical fitness. The athlete who wants to optimize his personal conditioning program should keep the following points in mind concerning multiple sets:

1. The same results could be obtained by performing fewer sets.

2. It is possible that greater results could be obtained by performing fewer sets.

3. Multiple sets performed by an athlete cannot be **properly** performed sets.

More often than not, the individual athlete who trains using multiple sets paces himself and saves his energy for the last set of an exercise. This is the set where he usually exerts his maximum effort. This is the set that will usually stimulate the greatest increase in strength. However, such an individual has wasted valuable time by performing the previous low-intensity sets.

## FREQUENCY OF WORKOUT

The **frequency of workout** is defined as the number of training sessions per week. It is recommended that an athlete exercise three times per week on alternate days. A muscle must be exercised every 48-72 hours or it will begin to atrophy, regardless of the individual's level of fitness. Even the muscles of a champion weightlifter or athlete will begin to atrophy if he does not exercise within 48-72 hours. On the other hand, a muscle requires 48-72 hours to adapt or fully recover from an exercise. This is the purpose for alternating days. Workouts performed on consecutive days will eventually do more harm than good. Daily workouts will eventually reach a point of diminishing returns because the body is no longer capable of adapting to the exercise. Figure 4-10 illustrates what happens to the level of strength of a muscle after exercise and during its recovery period before the next workout.

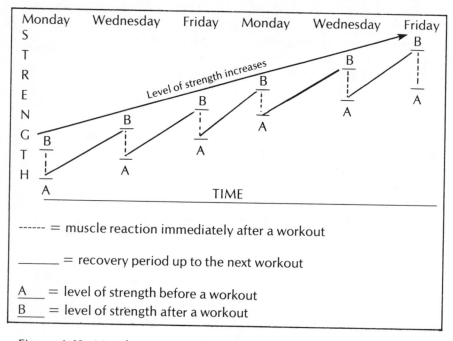

Figure 4-10. Muscle recovery patterns before and after alternate day workouts.

As can be observed, the strength level of a muscle is lower immediately after a workout. An individual is not as strong immediately after a workout as he was before the workout. The gain in strength takes place during the recovery period **between** workouts.

A muscle will continue to gain strength if two things occur. First, it must be forced to work harder during each successive workout. And second, it must be given adequate time to recover before the next workout (48-72 hrs.). A gain in strength should be observed (regardless of how small) each and every workout. If the athlete has had adequate food, sleep, etc., and he still does not record an increase in strength each workout, he must assume that one or more of the following is probably taking place.

1. He is performing too much exercise.
2. He is not allowing adequate time for his body to recover.
3. The intensity of his exercise is too low to stimulate an increase in your strength.

Figure 4-11 illustrates what happens to the strength level of a muscle if it is exercised daily (which does not allow the muscle adequate time to recover between workouts).

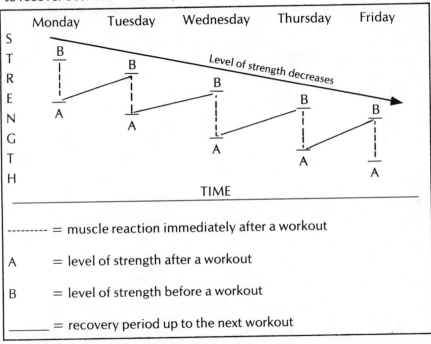

Figure 4-11. Muscle recovery patterns before and after daily workouts.

**Do not fall into the training cycle utilized by far too many athletes— hard work, little rest, and more hard work. Hard work in moderation is the key to any exercise program if the muscles are given time to rest and adapt to the stresses of the previous workout.**

## EXERCISES TO BE PERFORMED

The **exercises to be performed** are the specific exercises which are used to meet individual needs and program objectives. There are a multitude of exercises from which to choose for each muscle or muscle group.

In order to determine which exercises should be used, the athlete should perform a simple mechanical analysis of his sport and decide which of his major muscle groups are involved. (In other words, the athlete should perform the movements related to his sport and observe which muscles he is actually using). Once you have identified the prime movers used in your sport you can choose a specific exercise to develop them. For example, let us consider a football player. It is obvious that the football player involves all of the major muscles of the body to play the game. He would, therefore, use exercises to develop all of the major muscles in the body.

Below is a sample workout that could be used by a football player when the only equipment available is conventional free weight equipment.

| Exercise | Prime Movers | Muscles Involved |
|---|---|---|
| Squat | Buttocks, quadriceps | Buttocks, quads, hams, calves |
| Leg extension | Quadriceps | Quadriceps |
| Leg curl | Hamstrings | Hamstrings |
| Heel raise | Calves | Calves |
| Bench press | Pectorals | Pectorals, deltoids, triceps |
| Bent arm pullover | Pectorals, latissimus | Pectorals, latissimus dorsi, biceps |
| Seated press | Deltoids | Deltoids, pectorals, triceps |
| Chinups | Latissimus dorsi | Latissimus dorsi, biceps |
| Dips | Triceps | Pectorals, deltoids, triceps |
| Biceps curl | Biceps | same |
| Wrist curl | Forearm flexors | same |
| Situps | Abdominals | Abdominals |
| Neck exercises | Neck muscles | same |

The equipment available will obviously affect the exercises to be performed. The method in selecting the exercises will remain the same, however. Analyze the movement, decide which muscles are being used, choose an exercise to develop those specific muscles. (Editor's note: the reader is referred to Chapter 13 for additional information on this aspect).

## ORDER OF EXERCISE

The **order of exercise** is one of the variables of a strength development program in which some degree of flexibility exists.

The body can be divided into five individual segments: (1) legs: (2) torso; (3) arms; (4) abdominals; and (5) neck. The largest and strongest muscle groups should be exercised first while progressing to the smaller and weaker muscles.

Since the hips and legs have the greatest potential for developing strength and muscle mass, they should be exercised first. When exercising the leg muscles, the order of the muscles being exercised should be as follows: (1) quadriceps - buttocks; (2) hamstrings; and (3) calves. The torso should be the next body segment to be exercised. There are two distinct movements in performing an exercise for the torso: either a pressing or pulling movement. Because an individual is limited to pressing and pulling movements when exercising the torso muscles, he should change the position of his body to effectively place the emphasis on a specific muscle or group of muscles. For example, the bench press, incline press, decline press, and seated press, are all pressing movements, but the emphasis is placed on different muscles or areas of the same muscle simply by changing the position of the body. When performing any pressing movement for the torso, the primary muscle groups exerting the effort are the pectorals, deltoids, and triceps. When executing a pulling movement for the torso, the primary muscles being employed are the latissimus dorsi and the biceps (exceptions are the bent-arm pullover and upright row).

In his workout when exercising the torso muscles, the athlete should alternate a pressing movement with a pulling movement. By alternating a pressing movement with the pulling movement, he allows the opposing muscle groups adequate time to recover before performing another exercise.

The arms should be exercised **after,** and **not before,** the much larger and stronger muscle groups of the torso. The muscles of the arms must be used to perform most of the exercises for the torso. To fatigue the smaller and weaker muscle groups of the arms first and then attempt to exercise the torso would provide very little benefit for the much larger and stronger torso muscles. When exercising the upper arm muscles (biceps-triceps), the athlete should perform either a pulling or a pressing movement (in which the triceps were used) the first exercise performed for the arms should be a pulling movement (for the biceps).

The forearms should be exercised after the biceps and triceps. The rationale here is that grip strength (forearm flexors) is needed to perform most of the exercises for the biceps and triceps.

Exercises for the abdominals should be performed after the completion of all exercises for the legs, torso, and arms. The physiological rationale here is that the abdominal muscles are used in most exercises to stabilize the rib cage and abdominal wall. If an individual performs a high intensity exercise for the abdominals first, they will become fatigued. This will not allow the athlete to exert a maximum effort on a subsequent exercise in which the abdominals are required to act as stabilizers. Few individuals have ever performed a properly executed set of situps which denies them the opportunity to perceive the discomfort that follows a properly executed set of situps.

The neck muscles should be exercised **last** because the muscles of the neck support the head. If these muscles are totally fatigued first, you will have difficulty in performing an exercise in which the neck muscles must support the head.

Admittedly, the "7 Variables" encompass an abundance of material for the beginning or novice lifter to remember when initiating his muscular development program. Since it is very difficult to recall all of the pertinent information that has been discussed about the organization of a program, the athlete should use a "program data sheet" (Figure 4-12) to provide him with an outline of the basic information of his progress. Eventually, the beginning lifter will become familiar with the workout data and need only to periodically check his data sheet to reinforce his training techniques.

## WORKLOAD

The **workload** is the amount of weight to be used when performing an exercise. For maximum gains in strength, the amount of weight should be that which will cause the athlete to reach the point of momentary muscular failure somewhere between 8 and 12 repetitions. Anything less than a maximum workload will produce less than maximum gains in strength and muscle mass. Keep in mind, however, it is **now how much** weight you lift that produces results but **how** you lift the weight that counts.

Many coaches and athletes become more concerned with **how much** weight is being lifted rather than **how** the weight is being lifted. Any deviation from the proper training techniques will result in less than maximum gains in strength. The athlete's primary objective in the weight room is to develop strength and not demonstrate it. The athlete

| Pounds | Letters | Colors |
|--------|---------|--------|
| 10 | A | Red |
| 20 | B | Green |
| 30 | C | Yellow |
| 40 | D | Blue |
| 50 | E | Orange |
| 60 | F | Brown |

should never sacrifice either form or technique to increase the amount of weight to be lifted.

For example, during one workout an athlete can properly perform 8 repetitions of the bench press exercise with 225 pounds but is unable to perform 9 repetitions. During the next workout, however, his coach is present, observing the athlete's performance. Obviously, the athlete will want to impress the coach with "how much" weight he can lift. During this "demonstration of strength" the athlete deemphasizes the lowering of the weight, bounces the weight off the chest, bridges while extending his arms, and various other methods of cheating. The athlete is using momentum and gravity to raise and lower the weight and he now performs 12 repetitions with the same weight. Even though more repetitions were performed by making the exercise easier, the lifter will benefit less. In addition, and perhaps most importantly, his chances of being injured will be increased.

One technique which can be used to minimize the athlete's preoccupation with "weight" is to replace the numbers on the weight stacks of the exercise machines with either letters or colored squares. The important point is that the alternate code should deemphasize the amount of weight being lifted (see diagrams below). Instead of recording 50 pounds, the athlete records either the letter or the color on his workout card to denote the number of plates being lifted.

The athlete should be somewhat cautious when selecting a starting weight for an exercise which he has not previously performed. Before engaging in an all out effort he should become very familiar with the proper execution of the exercise. Once he has accomplished this, he should then select a starting weight which will allow him to properly execute at least 10 repetitions. During each succeeding workout, he should gradually increase the weight until he is exerting a maximum effort and is reaching the point of momentary muscular failure somewhere between 8 and 12 repetitions. When he can perform 12 properly executed repetitions of an exercise, he should then increase the weight by five to ten pounds. The athlete should then exercise with this new weight until he once again can perform 12 repetitions. At this point he again increases the weight by five to ten pounds.

## TIME INTERVAL BETWEEN EXERCISES

The **time interval between exercises** (or sets) is the amount of time elapsed between exercises. If the athlete uses a barbell to perform two sets of the **same** exercise, very little time to recover between sets should be allowed (for maximum efficiency). The athlete should only allow

## SAMPLE PROGRAM DATA SHEET

Equipment available _____ Universal Gym _____

Number of repetitions to be executed _____ Between 8 and 12 _____

Number of sets to be performed __1__

Workload _____ Enough so that you fail momentarily between 8 and 12 reps _____

Time Interval
    between sets _____ N/A _____
    between exercises _____ 1 minute _____

Frequency of workout _____ Monday - Wednesday - Friday _____

| **Order** of the **exercises** to be performed | Primary Muscle Groups |
|---|---|
| 1. Leg press | Buttocks, legs |
| 2. Leg extension | Quadriceps |
| 3. Leg curl | Hamstrings |
| 4. Bench press | Pectorals, deltoids, triceps |
| 5. Chins | Latissimus dorsi, biceps |
| 6. Seated press | Pectorals, deltoids, triceps |
| 7. Lat pulldowns | Latissimus dorsi, biceps |
| 8. Dips | Pectorals, deltoids, triceps |
| 9. Biceps curls | Biceps |
| 10. Situps - leg raises | Abdominals |

**Points to emphasize**
1. Exercise through the muscle's full range of movement.
2. Use proper techniques when performing all exercises.
3. Emphasize quality exercise, not total quantity of weight lifted.
4. Observe the overload principle—you must try to lift more weight; perform more repetitions; or both.
5. Monitor each workout—record all pertinent information—the amount of weight, the number of repetitions, the date, etc.
6. Periodically evaluate your progress.

Figure 4-12. Sample program data sheet.

enough time to make a weight change and then immediately perform the second set.

The time interval between two **different** exercises may vary depending upon the objective of the program. In a strength development program which is also designed to increase cardiorespiratory fitness, the time interval between exercises should be as brief as possible. The athlete should move from one exercise to the next as quickly as possible, minimizing recovery time from the previous exercise.

In a program designed to increase strength only, as much time as is needed to adequately recover from one exercise before going on to the next exercise should be allowed. An athlete has recovered adequately from the previous exercise when you can again exert a maximum effort while performing an exercise.

# CHAPTER 5
## Free Weight Exercises

Daniel P. Riley
Director of Strength Training

Chapter Format
Exercises for the legs and buttocks
Exercises for the torso
Exercises for the arm
Exercises for the abdominals
Exercises for the neck

A properly organized muscular development program will include at least one exercise to develop each of the major muscles within the body. The selection of a particular exercise for a specific muscle group depends upon the equipment available and the individual lifter's personal preference.

The athlete who is limited by either time or equipment to performing only one exercise for each of the body's major muscle groups should perform a **core** exercise for each group. A **core** exercise is a lift which is designed to effectively isolate and develop a specific muscle or muscle group. Whenever prudent, a **supplementary** exercise can be substituted for a core exercise. Periodic varying of the exercises which are included in the program not only adds variety to the training regimen, but also provides the lifter with the opportunity to achieve developmental benefits not present in the regular program.


CHAPTER FORMAT

All of the most commonly performed exercises which use either free weights or Universal machines are described in this chapter. The exercises are grouped according to which area of the body is developed (legs and buttocks, torso, arm, abdominals, and neck). For each exercise, the following format is used:

# Exercise: The name of the exercise is listed.

a. **Equipment:** The equipment needed to perform the exercise is listed.

b. **Muscles Used:** The major muscles used to perform the exercise are listed.

c. **Prime Mover:** The prime mover or the primary muscle required to perform the exercise is listed.

d. **Starting Position:** A brief description of the starting position emphasizing the body position, stance, location of the bar or apparatus, etc.

e. **Description:** The execution of one repetition is described.

f. **Breathing:** The breathing pattern for one repetition is described. The recommended breathing pattern is designed to provide maximum efficiency while executing each repetition.

g. **Spotting:** The responsibilities of the spotter are outlined.

h. **Points to Emphasize:** Any additional information that could facilitate the proper execution or safety of the exercise is listed.

## EXERCISES FOR THE LEGS AND BUTTOCKS

1. **Exercise:** Squat (Fig. 5-1 and 5-2)

a. **Equipment:** Barbell, squat racks

b. **Muscles Used:** Major muscles of the legs, buttocks

c. **Prime Mover:** Buttocks, quadriceps

d. **Starting Position:** Standing with feet approximately shoulder width apart, barbell resting on trapezius and posterior deltoids.

e. **Description:** Lower the buttocks until the thighs are at least parallel to the floor, pause momentarily and recover to the starting position.

f. **Breathing:** Inhale when lowering to the squatting position and exhale upon recovery to the starting position.

g. **Spotting:** (Fig. 5-3) the spotter should stand behind the lifter as close as possible to him without interfering with the lift. If the lifter needs assistance in recovering to the starting position the spotter should place his arms around the lifter's chest and pull up until the lifter is in the upright position. This will prevent the lifter from folding at the waist and possibly injuring the lower back.

h. **Points to Emphasize:**

(1) Look upward when performing the exercise.

(2) Try to keep the bar in line with the base of support (the feet).

(3) Eliminate any bouncing during the squatting portion of the exercise (such bouncing can damage the knee joint).

2. **Exercise:** Leg Press (Fig. 5-4 and 5-5)

a. **Equipment:** Universal gym

b. **Muscles Used:** Major muscles of the leg, buttocks

c. **Prime Mover:** Buttocks, quadriceps

d. **Starting Position:** Seated with the feet on the leg press pedals, grasp the side of the seat with the hands.

e. **Description:** Extend the legs, pause momentarily and recover to the starting position.

f. **Breathing:** Inhale while recovering to the starting position and

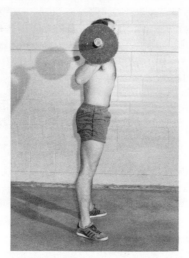

Figure 5-1. The starting position for the **squat**.

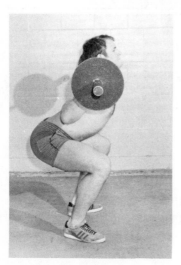

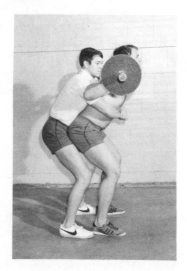

Figure 5-2. Execution of the **squat**.     Figure 5-3. Spotting for the **squat**.

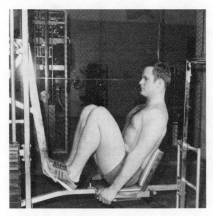

Figure 5-4. Starting
position for the **leg press.**

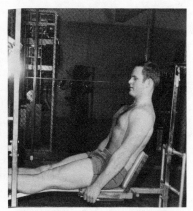

Figure 5-5. Execution
of the **leg press.**

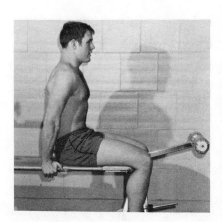

Figure 5-6. Starting
position for the **leg extension.**

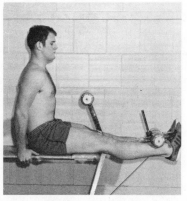

Figure 5-7. Execution
of the **leg extension.**

exhale when the legs are extended.

g. **Spotting:** N/A

h. **Points to Emphasize:**

(1) Pull downward with the hands to keep the buttocks in contact with the seat.

(2) Do not allow the legs to lock out (this allows the muscles to recover momentarily).

(3) Adjust the seat so that you are exercising through range of movement needed to perform your particular activity.


3. **Exercise:** Leg Extension (Fig. 5-6 and 5-7)

a. **Equipment:** Leg extension machine

b. **Muscles Used:** Quadriceps

c. **Prime Mover:** Quadriceps

d. **Starting Position:** Sitting on the extension machine, leaning back slightly, hands grasping the sides of the machine.

e. **Description:** Extend the legs until they are completely extended, pause momentarily, recover to the starting position.

f. **Breathing:** Inhale while lowering the weight and exhale when raising the weight.

g. **Spotting:** N/A

h. **Points to Emphasize:**

(1) Do not raise the buttocks off the bench when the weight is being lowered.

(2) Pause momentarily in the legs extended position (eliminate any bouncing movements).


4. **Exercise:** Leg Curl (Fig. 5-8 and 5-9)

a. **Equipment:** Leg curl machine

b. **Muscles Used:** Hamstrings

c. **Prime Mover:** Hamstrings

d. **Starting Position:** Lying face down on the leg curl machine with the heels hooked under the pads or rollers, the kneecaps should be just off the edge of the pad for maximum comfort.

e. **Description:** Flex the lower legs until they are at least perpendicular to the floor, pause momentarily and recover to the starting position.

f. **Breathing:** Inhale when raising the weight and exhale while lowering the weight.

g. **Spotting:** N/A

h. **Point to Emphasize:** Raise the weight so that the lower legs are at least perpendicular to the floor.

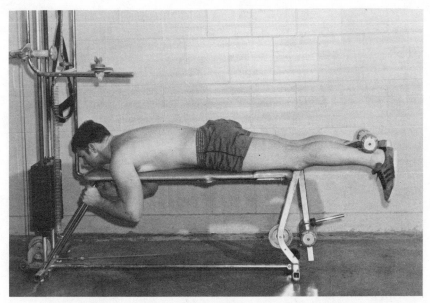

Figure 5-8. The starting position for the **leg curl**.

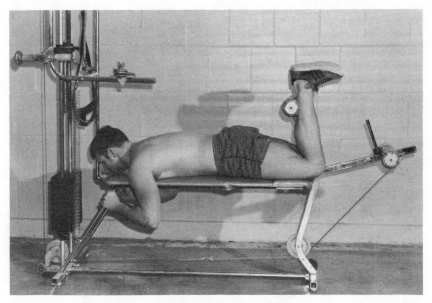

Figure 5-9. Execution of the **leg curl**.

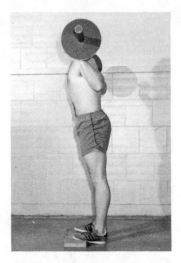

Figure 5-10. Starting position for the **heel raise** with a barbell.

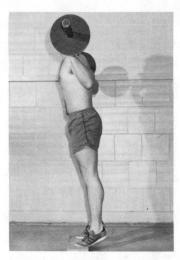

Figure 5-11. Execution of the **heel raise** with a barbell.

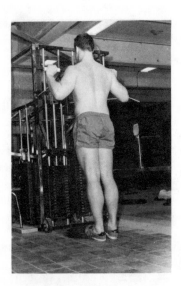

Figure 5-12. Starting position for the **heel raise** on a Universal machine.

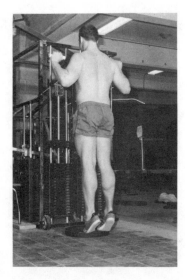

Figure 5-13. Execution of the **heel raise** on a Universal machine.

5. **Exercise:** Heel Raise
   a. **Equipment:** Barbell (Fig. 5-10 and 5-11), or Universal (Fig. 5-12 and 5-13).
   b. **Muscles Used:** Calves
   c. **Prime Mover:** Calves
   d. **Starting Position:** Standing with a barbell across the shoulders, toes should be elevated to provide maximum stretching.
   e. **Description:** Raise the heels off the floor while rising up on the toes, pause and slowly recover to the starting position.
   f. **Breathing:** Normal
   g. **Spotting:** N/A
   h. **Points to Emphasize:**
   (1) Elevate the heel as high as possible each repetition.
   (2) Raise the weight slowly and emphasize the lowering of the weight.

## EXERCISES FOR THE TORSO

1. **Exercise:** Bench Press
   a. **Equipment:** Exercise bench with standards, barbell (fig. 5-14 and 5-15) or Universal Gym (Fig. 5-16 and 5-17)
   b. **Muscles Used:** Pectorals, deltoids, triceps
   c. **Prime Mover:** Pectorals
   d. **Starting Position:** Lay face up on an exercise bench with the knees bent and the feet flat on the floor, the buttocks and shoulder blades are in contact with the bench, the barbell is in the arms extended position.
   e. **Description:** Lower the barbell to the chest, pause momentarily and recover to the starting position.
   f. **Breathing:** Inhale when lowering the weight and exhale while recovering to the starting position.
   g. **Spotting** (Fig. 5-18): The spotter should assist the lifter into the starting position. If the lifter is unable to complete a repetition the spotter will assist him only as much as is needed to complete the repetition. The lifter will need assistance when the bar is nearest the chest. The spotter would be bent at the waist with the hands **under** the bar and **not over** it.
   h. **Points to Emphasize:**
   (1) Do not arch the back. This could provide a mechanical advantage but may cause injury to the lower back.
   (2) The lifter should lower the bar to the chest each repetition touching the chest at the same spot, without bouncing the bar, and maintaining eye contact with the bar throughout.
   (3) With the arms vertical to the floor the barbell should be lowered to the chest in a straight line.

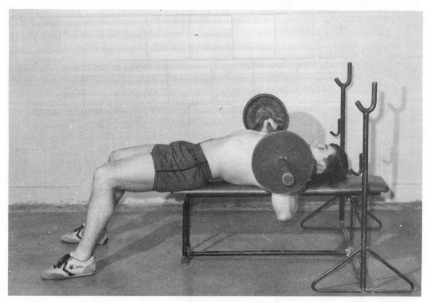

Figure 5-14. Starting position for the **bench press** with a barbell.

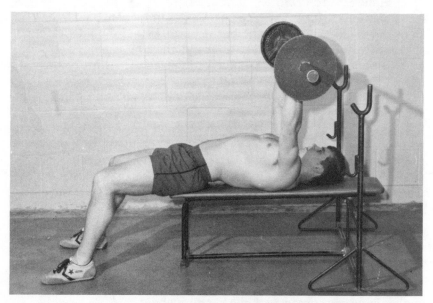

Figure 5-15. Execution of the **bench press** with a barbell.

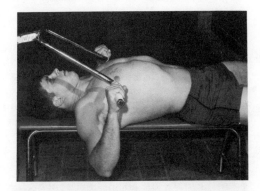

Figure 5-16. Starting position for the **bench press** on a Universal machine.

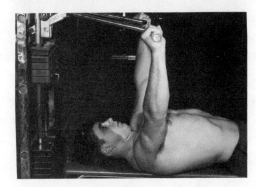

Figure 5-17. Execution of the **bench press** on a Universal machine.

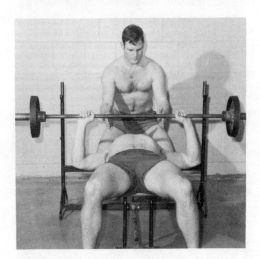

Figure 5-18. Spotting for the **bench press.**

(4) When recovering to the starting position the barbell is pressed upward and slightly backward so that upon completion of the repetition the barbell is approximately over the neck (a readjustment to the vertical position is necessary before initiating the next repetition).

(5) Injury to the shoulder may occur if 3 and 4 above are not observed.

(6) Dumbbells may be used to perform this exercise.

2. **Exercise:** Incline Press
   a. **Equipment:** Incline bench, barbell (fig. 5-19 and 5-20) or dumbbells (Fig. 5-21 and 5-22)
   b. **Muscles Used:** Pectorals, deltoids, triceps
   c. **Prime Mover:** Pectorals (emphasis placed on the upper region of the pectorals)
   d. **Starting Position:** Lying on the back on an incline bench with a barbell or dumbbells in the arms extended position.
   e. **Description:** Lower the weight to the top of the rib cage and recover to the arms extended position.
   f. **Breathing:** Inhale when lowering the bar and exhale when recovering to the arms extended position.
   g. **Spotting:** The spotter may stand to the rear of the lifter giving assistance when needed by placing the hands on the lifter's wrist (this will allow the spotter to assist the lifter in maintaining control of the bar or dumbbell).
   h. **Points to Emphasize:**
   (1) Dumbbells (if used) should be held so that the palms are facing **away** from the body.
   (2) As you fatigue the tendency will be for the dumbbells to fall away from the center of the body; therefore, when extending the arms you should bring the dumbbells together in the arms extended position.
   (3) Lower the bar so that it remains perpendicular to the floor (not the body).

3. **Exercise:** Decline Press
   a. **Equipment:** Decline bench, barbell or dumbbells
   b. **Muscles Used:** Pectorals, deltoids, triceps
   c. **Prime Mover:** Pectorals (emphasis is placed on the lower region of the pectorals).
   d. **Starting Position:** Lying on the back on a decline bench with the barbell or dumbbells in the arms extended position.
   e. **Description:** Lower the bar to the lower part of the chest and then recover to the arms extended position.
   f. **Breathing:** Inhale when the weight is lowered and exhale while

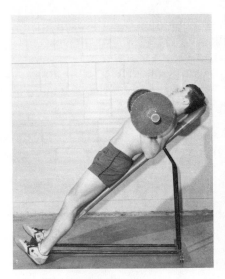

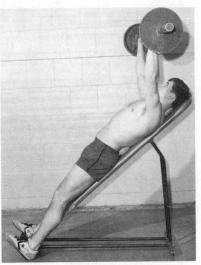

Figure 5-19. Starting position for the **incline press** with a barbell.

Figure 5-20. Execution of the **incline press** with a barbell.

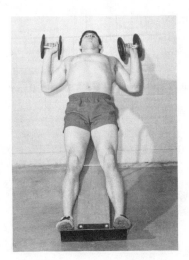

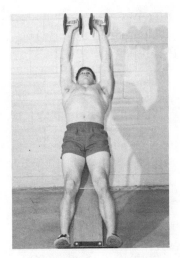

Figure 5-21. Starting position for the **incline press** with dumbells.

Figure 5-22. Execution of the **incline press** with dumbells.

recovering to the starting position.

g. **Spotting:** The spotter will stand behind the lifter assisting him by placing his hands on the lifter's wrist.

h. **Points to Emphasize:**

(1) Lower the bar so that it remains perpendicular to the floor.

(2) Bring dumbbells together in the arms extended position.

(3) Lower the dumbbells simultaneously.

4. **Exercise:** Bent Arm Flies (Fig. 5-23 and 5-24)

a. **Equipment:** Exercise bench, incline or decline bench

b. **Muscles Used:** Pectorals

c. **Starting Position:** Lying on the back on a bench with the arms extended in a semi-flexed position.

d. **Description:** Lower the dumbbells downward and sideward while maintaining the semi-flexed position of the arms and then recover to the starting position.

e. **Breathing:** Inhale while lowering the weight and exhale when recovering to the starting position.

f. **Spotting:** N/A

g. **Points to Emphasize:**

(1) Keep the arms locked in a semi-flexed position.

(2) Allow the pectorals to be stretched maximally when the weight is being lowered.

5. **Exercise:** Bent Arm Pullover (Fig. 5-25 and 5-26)

a. **Equipment:** Exercise bench, barbell or dumbbells

b. **Muscles Used:** Pectorals, lattissimus dorsi, biceps, intercostals (muscles between the ribs).

c. **Prime Mover:** Rib cage (emphasis is placed on the overall development of the rib cage).

d. **Starting Position:** Lay face up on an exercise bench, back flat, with the neck extended over the edge of the bench so that the **top** of the head is parallel to the floor; the feet may be hooked around the legs of the bench to prevent the lifter from being pulled off the bench; the barbell should be resting at the top of the rib cage just above the neck.

e. **Description:** Lower the bar toward the floor letting the barbell come as close as possible to the forehead and chin as it passes by, and then recover to the starting position.

f. **Breathing:** Inhale while lowering the weight and exhale when recovering to the starting position.

g. **Spotting:** Hand the barbell to the lifter so that the bar is resting on the chest; the lifter may elect to complete the exercise with the barbell on the floor or in the starting position. If the lifter finishes the exercise

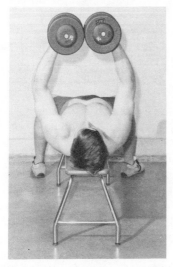

Figure 5-23. Starting position for the **bent arm fly.**

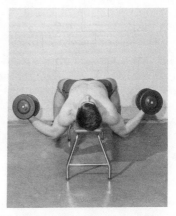

Figure 5-24. Execution of the **bent arm fly.**

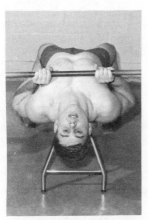

Figure 5-25. Starting position for the **bent arm pullover.**

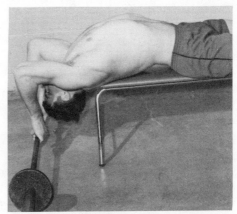

Figure 5-26. Execution of the **bent arm pullover.**

in the starting position the spotter will place the barbell on the floor.

6. **Exercise:** Seated Press
   a. **Equipment:** Barbell (Fig. 5-27 and 5-28) or Universal Gym (Fig. 5-29 and 5-30)
   b. **Muscles Used:** Deltoids, triceps
   c. **Prime Mover:** Deltoids
   d. **Starting Position:** Seated on an exercise bench with the barbell resting on the shoulders, behind the neck, feet should be hooked on the bench legs to prevent the lifter from falling backwards.
   e. **Description:** Raise the weight so that the arms become momentarily extended and recover to the starting position.
   f. **Breathing:** Inhale while the weight is being lowered and exhale when raising the weight.
   g. **Spotting:** Behind the lifter to assist him in raising the weight if necessary.
   h. **Points to Emphasize:**
      (1) Lower the barbell completely so that it touches the base of the neck (each repetition).
      (2) Do not lean back when extending the arms; this is a form of cheating. The weight you are using is too heavy and you are trying to recruit the pectorals to assist. It also places undue stress on the lower back.
      (3) Dumbbells may be used. If dumbbells are used it is suggested that they be raised and lowered alternately.

7. **Exercise:** Upright Row
   a. **Equipment:** Barbell (Fig. 5-31 and 5-32) or Universal Gym (Fig. 5-33 and 5-34)
   b. **Muscles Used:** Deltoids, biceps, trapezius
   c. **Prime Mover:** Deltoids
   d. **Starting Position:** Standing with the arms extended downward with the barbell in both hands, a closer than shoulder width grip should be used, feet shoulder width apart.
   e. **Description:** Pull the barbell upward touching the bar with the chin, pause momentarily and recover to the starting position.
   f. **Breathing:** Inhale while raising the weight and exhale when recovering to the starting position.
   g. **Spotting:** N/A
   h. **Points to Emphasize:**
      (1) Do not bend at the waist (stand perfectly straight).
      (2) Raise and lower the bar in a straight line.
      (3) Let the shoulder girdle relax when the arms are completely extended.

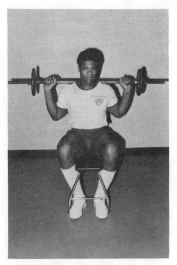

Figure 5-27. Starting position for the **seated press** with a barbell.

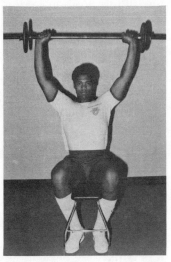

Figure 5-28. Execution of the **seated press** with a barbell.

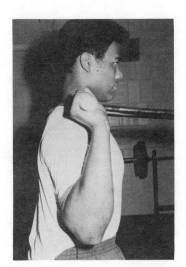

Figure 5-29. Starting position for the **seated press** on a Universal machine.

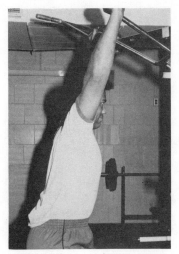

Figure 5-30. Execution of the **seated press** on a Universal machine.

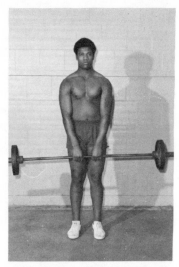

Figure 5-31. Starting position for the **upright row** with a barbell.

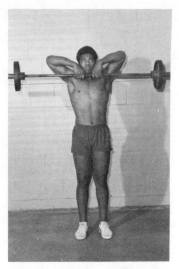

Figure 5-32. Execution of the **upright row** with a barbell.

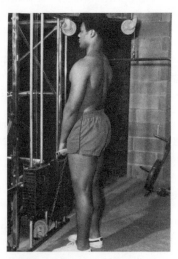

Figure 5-33. Starting position for the **upright row** on a Universal machine.

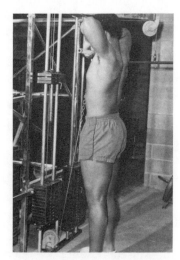

Figure 5-34. Execution of the **upright row** on a Univeral machine.

8. **Exercise:** Side Lateral Raises (Fig. 5-35 and 5-36)
   a. **Equipment:** Dumbbells
   b. **Muscles Used:** Deltoids
   c. **Prime Mover:** Deltoids
   d. **Starting Position:** Standing with the arms extended downward, palms facing each other with the dumbbells touching in front of the body, the body is slightly bent forward at the waist.
   e. **Description:** Raise the dumbbells sideward and upward so that the dumbbells are approximately parallel with the head, pause momentarily and recover to the starting position.
   f. **Breathing:** Inhale while raising the weight and exhale when lowering the weight.
   g. **Spotting:** A spotter can apply resistance (manually) to the lifter's hands while he raises his arms sideward and upward (this will eliminate the need for using dumbells).

9. **Exercise:** Dead Lift (Fig. 5-37 and 5-38)
   a. **Equipment:** Barbell
   b. **Muscles Used:** Lower back, buttocks, legs
   c. **Prime Mover:** Lower back
   d. **Starting Position:** Assume a semi-squatting position keeping the head up and the back straight, feet should be approximately shoulder width apart; grasp the barbell with an alternate grip.
   e. **Description:** Stand to an erect position keeping the arms extended and recover to the starting position.
   f. **Breathing:** Inhale while raising the weight and exhale when recovering to the starting position.
   g. **Spotting:** N/A
   h. **Points to Emphasize:**
   (1) More emphasis will be placed on the lower back by performing a stifflegged deadlift (Fig. 5-39 and 5-40). The feet can be elevated so that maximum stretching will be provided when the weight is lowered (also use smaller barbell plates).

10. **Exercise:** Good Morning (Fig. 5-41 and 5-42)
    a. **Equipment:** Barbell
    b. **Muscles Used:** Lower back
    c. **Prime Mover:** Lower back
    d. **Starting Position:** Standing with the barbell behind the neck resting on the shoulders, feet spread shoulder width apart, legs locked.
    e. **Description:** Bend forward at the waist until the body is below

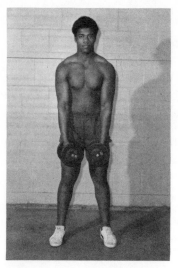

Figure 5-35. Starting position for the **side lateral raise.**

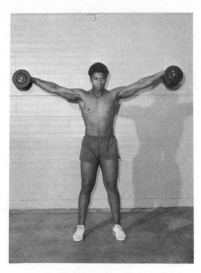

Figure 5-36. Execution of the **side lateral raise.**

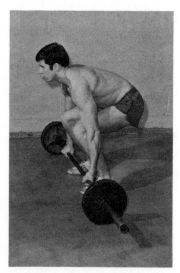

Figure 5-37. Starting position for the **dead lift.**

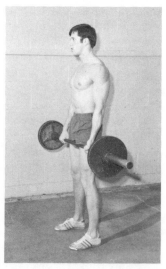

Figure 5-38. Execution of the **dead lift.**

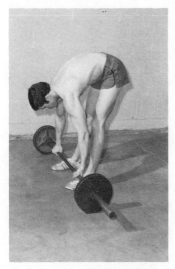

Figure 5-39. Starting
position for the
**stifflegged dead lift.**

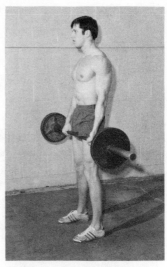

Figure 5-40. Execution
of the **stifflegged dead lift.**

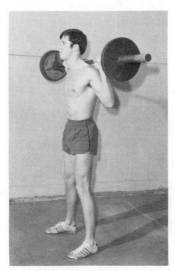

Figure 5-41. Starting
position for the
**good morning.**

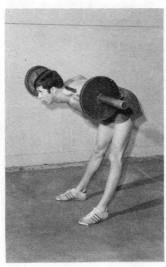

Figure 5-42. Execution of
the **good morning.**

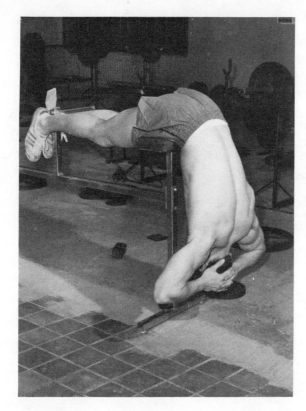

Figure 5-43.
Starting position
for the
**hyperextension.**

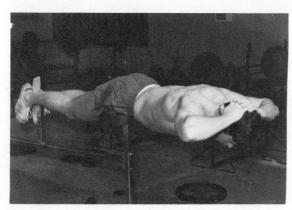

Figure 5-44.
Execution of the
**hyperextension.**

parallel with the floor, pause momentarily and recover to the starting position.

f. **Breathing:** Inhale while lowering the weight and exhale when recovering to the starting position.

g. **Spotting:** N/A

h. **Suggestions:** Keep the head up at all times.

11. **Exercise:** Hyper Extension (Fig. 5-43 and 5-44)

a. **Equipment:** Bench or table three to four feet high or Universal hyper extention station

b. **Muscles Used:** Lower back

c. **Prime Mover:** Lower back

d. **Starting Position:** Lying face down with the legs and hips on the bench with the upper body bent forward hanging over the bench so that the upper body is perpendicular to the floor, hands should be interlocked behind the head.

e. **Description:** Raise the body forward and upward until the body is parallel to the floor, "pause momentarily" and recover to the starting position.

f. **Breathing:** Inhale while raising the weight and exhale when recovering to the starting position.

g. **Spotting:** The spotter will hold the lifter's legs down on the bench so that he will not fall off.

h. **Points to Emphasize:**

(1) The initial starting weight is fixed (the weight of your torso). This starting weight may be too heavy for your lower back muscles. Be cautious!

(2) Eliminate any bouncing movements when raising the weights.

(3) Do not hyperextend the back (could cause lower back injury).

(4) Additional weight can be added by holding a weight behind the head.

12. **Exercise:** Bent Over Rowing

a. **Equipment:** Barbell (Fig. 5-45 and 5-46) or dumbbell (Fig. 5-47 and 5-48)

b. **Muscles Used:** Latissimus dorsi, biceps

c. **Prime Mover:** Latissimus dorsi

d. **Starting Position:** Standing with the body bent forward at the waist so that the upper body is parallel to the floor, feet shoulder width apart, knees slightly flexed (to take the pressure off the lower back).

e. **Description:** Pull the barbell upward so that the barbell touches the chest, pause momentarily and recover to the starting position.

f. **Breathing:** Inhale while raising the weight and exhale when lower-

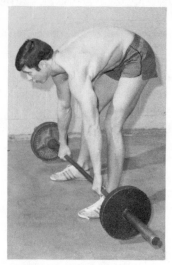

Figure 5-45. Starting position for the **bent over rowing** with a barbell.

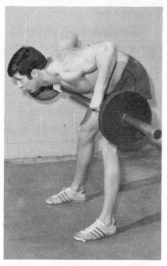

Figure 5-46. Execution of the **bent over rowing** with a barbell.

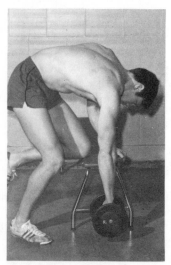

Figure 5-47. Starting position for the **bent over rowing** with dumbell.

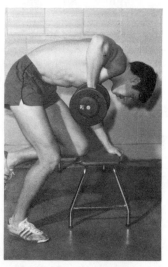

Figure 5-48. Execution of the **bent over rowing** with a dumbell.

ing the weight to the starting position.

   g. **Spotting:** N/A

   h. **Points to Emphasize:**

     (1) A bench may be used to rest the forehead upon, this will stabilize the body in the bent over position.

     (2) Keep the back of the hand on top of the bar (do not flex wrists)

     (3) Do not pull the weight toward the stomach. The bar should travel in a line that is perpendicular to the floor.

     (4) An inefficient exercise for the lats, the biceps will fail first (you will not be able to pull the bar all the way up to the chest.)

     (6) A seated row on the Universal may be performed to duplicate the bent over row with a barbell (performed at the biceps curl station).

13.   **Exercise:** Lat Pulldowns, with overhand grip (Fig. 5-49 and 5-50)

   a. **Equipment:** Lat machine or lat machine on Universal Gym

   b. **Muscles Used:** Latissimus dorsi

   c. **Prime Mover:** Latissimus dorsi

   d. **Starting Position:** Assume a kneeling or seated position on the floor so that the back of the neck is directly under the bar on the lat machine.

   e. **Description:** Using an overhand grip pull the bar downward to a position at the base of the neck, pause momentarily and recover to the starting position.

   f. **Breathing:** Inhale while pulling the bar downward and exhale when recovering to the starting position.

   g. **Spotting:** A spotter may be needed to apply pressure to the lifter's shoulders to prevent him from lifting off the floor; a weight may be strapped around the waist if a spotter is not available.

   h. **Points to Emphasize:**

     (1) Do not bend forward at the waist when pulling the weight downward.

     (2) Lower the weight slowly.

14.   **Exercise:** Lat Pulldown, with an underhand grip (Fig. 5-51 and 5-52).

   a. **Equipment:** Lat Machine

   b. **Muscles Used:** Latissimus dorsi, biceps

   c. **Prime Mover:** Latissimus dorsi

   d. **Starting Position:** Assume a kneeling or seated position using an underhand and shoulder width grip to grasp the bar.

   e. **Description:** Pull the bar downward and backward until the bar touches the "upper chest", pause momentarily and recover to the starting position.

   f. **Breathing:** Inhale when pulling the bar downward and exhale when

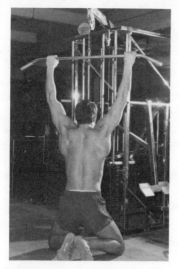

Figure 5-49. Starting position for the **lat pulldown** using an overhand grip.

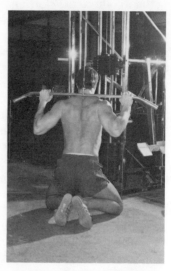

Figure 5-50. Execution of the **lat pulldown** using an overhand grip.

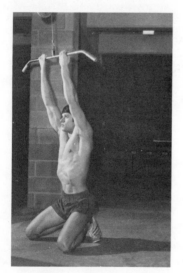

Figure 5-51. Starting position for the **lat pulldown** using an underhand grip.

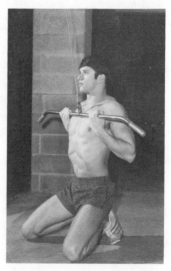

Figure 5-52. Execution of the **lat pulldown** using an underhand grip.

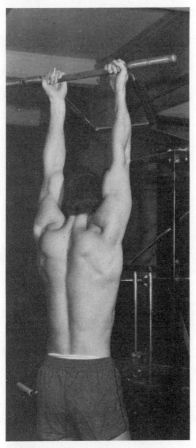 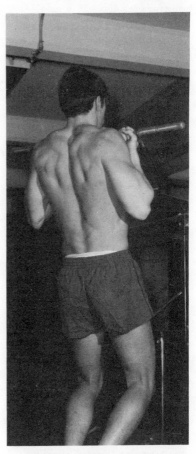

Figure 5-53. Starting position for the **chinup**.

Figure 5.54 Execution of the **chinup**.

recovering to the starting position.

g. **Spotting:** A spotter may be needed to prevent the lifter from lifting off the floor or chair. The spotter will apply pressure to the shoulders of the lifter.

h. **Points to Emphasize:**

When pulling the weight backward and downward, try to imagine that the elbows are pushing a weight backwards.

15. **Exercise:** Chinup (Fig. 5-53 and 5-54)

a. **Equipment:** Chin bar

b. **Muscles Used:** Latissimus dorsi, biceps

c. **Starting Position:** Hanging from a chinup bar with an underhand grip, the arms should be extended.

d. **Description:** Pull the body upward so that the chin is resting over the bar.

e. **Breathing:** Inhale while pulling the body upward and exhale when recovering to the starting position.

f. **Points to Emphasize:**

(1) To increase strength and mass most efficiently use an underhand grip.

(2) Do not use a wider than shoulder grip (the range of movement of the lats will be decreased).

(3) Emphasize the lowering of the body.

(4) Negative only chinups can be performed (a stool or steps are needed so that you can climb up and only lower the body weight).

16. **Exercise:** Shrugs

a. **Equipment:** Barbell (Fig. 5-55 and 5-56), Universal Machine (Fig. 5-57 and 5-58)

b. **Muscles Used:** Trapezius

c. **Prime Mover:** Trapezius

d. **Starting Position:** Standing with the arms extended with a barbell in hand, the shoulder girdle is relaxed.

e. **Description:** Elevate the shoulder girdle as high as possible, pause momentarily and recover to the starting position.

f. **Spotting:** N/A

g. **Points to Emphasize:**

(1) Do not bend the arms when raising the weight.

(2) The shoulder girdle should be completely relaxed in the starting position.

c. The exercise can be performed with a dumbbell in each hand.

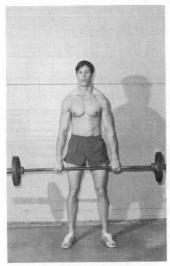

Figure 5-55. Starting position for the **shrug** with a barbell.

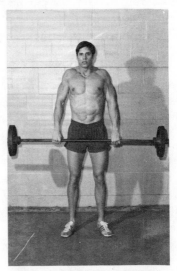

Figure 5-56. Execution of the **shrug** with a barbell.

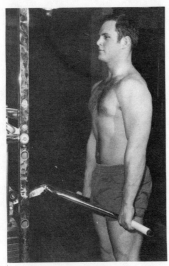

Figure 5-57. Starting position for the **shrug** on a Universal machine.

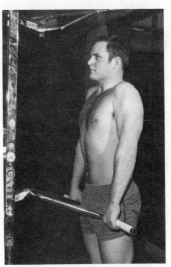

Figure 5-58. Execution of the **shrug** on a Universal machine.

## EXERCISES FOR THE ARM

1. **Exercise:** French Curl (Fig. 5-59 and 5-60)
   a. **Equipment:** Barbell, exercise bench
   b. **Muscles Used:** Triceps
   c. **Prime Mover:** Triceps
   d. **Starting Position:** Lying on the back on an exercise bench with the feet flat on the floor, the barbell is in the arms extended position with the arms vertical to the floor.
   e. **Description:** Bending only at the elbow, lower the barbell to the forehead and recover to the starting position. Fig. 5-61 illustrates a subject bending at the shoulder, an incorrect technique.
   f. **Breathing:** Inhale while lowering the weight and exhale when recovering to the starting position.
   g. **Spotting:** The spotter should hand the barbell to the lifter assisting him into the starting position. Upon completion of the exercise the spotter should replace the barbell to the floor.
   h. **Points to Emphasize:**
   (1) The upper arm should remain vertical to the floor.
   (2) Keep the elbows at shoulder width.
   (3) The exercise may be performed seated (very difficult to keep the elbows in and the upper arm perpendicular to the floor (Fig. 5-62).

2. **Exercise:** Triceps extension (on the lat machine)
   a. **Equipment:** Lat machine or Universal lat machine station (Fig. 5-63 and 5-64)
   b. **Muscle Used:** Triceps
   c. **Prime Mover:** Triceps
   d. **Starting Position:** Standing facing the bar with the lat bar pulled down to neck level, the elbows should be fixed to the rib cage. An overhand grip on the bar is used.
   e. **Description:** Moving only the lower arm press the weight downward until the arms are extended, pause momentarily and recover to the starting position.
   f. **Breathing:** Inhale while extending the arms and exhale when recovering to the starting position.
   g. **Spotting:** N/A
   h. **Points to Emphasize:**
   (1) Once the exercise has begun the elbows must remain fixed to the rib cage. Subject in Fig. 5-65 allows his elbows to move from his rib cage, which is an incorrect technique.
   (2) Do not bend forward at the waist (the body is trying to compensate by recruiting the pectorals).

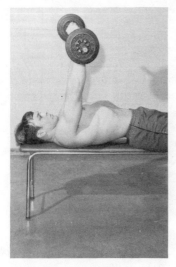

Figure 5-59. Starting position for a **french curl.**

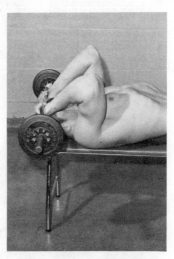

Figure 5-60. Execution of the **french curl.**

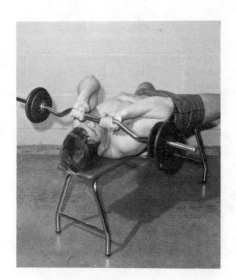

Figure 5-61. Incorrect technique for performing the **french curl.**

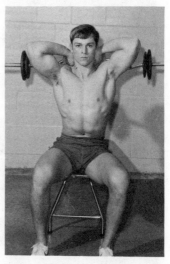

Figure 5-62. Starting position for the **french curl** from a seated position.

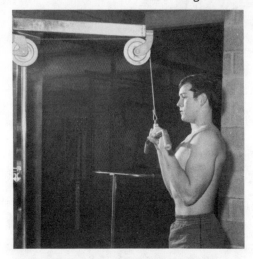

Figure 5-63. Starting position for the **triceps extension.**

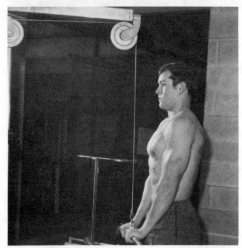

Figure 5-64. Execution of the **triceps extension.**

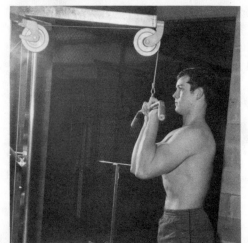

Figure 5-65. Incorrect technique for performing the **triceps extension.**

3. **Exercise:** Dips (Fig. 5-66 and 5-67)
   a. **Equipment:** Dip bars
   b. **Muscles Used:** Pectorals, deltoids, triceps
   c. **Prime Mover:** Triceps
   d. **Starting Position:** Mounted on the dip bars with the arms extended.
   e. **Description:** Bend the arms lowering the body as much as possible, pause momentarily and recover to the starting position.
   f. **Breathing:** Inhale while lowering the bodyweight and exhale when recovering to the starting position.
   g. **Spotting:** N/A
   h. **Points to Emphasize:**
   (1) Bend the knees so that a full range of movement can be obtained while lowering the body.
   (2) Additional weight should be added to the body once the lifter can perform 12 properly executed repetitions.
   (3) Lower the body slowly (4 seconds).
   (4) This exercise can be performed negative only (a stool or steps will be needed to raise the body).

4. **Exercise:** L-seat dips (Fig. 5-68 and 5-69)
   a. **Equipment:** Two exercise benches
   b. **Muscles Used:** Pectorals, deltoids, triceps
   c. **Prime Mover:** Triceps
   d. **Starting Position:** The body should be positioned between two exercise benches with the hands placed on one (shoulder width apart) and the heels of the feet on the other; the arms and legs are extended; the body is in an "L" position.
   e. **Description:** Bend the arms, lowering the body as far as possible; pause momentarily and recover to the starting position.
   f. **Breathing:** Inhale while lowering the body and exhale when recovering to the starting position.
   g. **Spotting:** Standing behind the lifter on the exercise bench with your hands on his shoulders, apply as much pressure as is needed to allow him to just barely complete 8-12 repetitions.
   h. **Points to Emphasize:**
   (1) When lowering the body, the back of the lifter should be as close as possible to the exercise bench.
   (2) The spotter must vary the resistance to accomodate the negative and positive part of the exercise (more pressure must be applied by the spotter when the lifter is lowering his bodyweight).

5. **Exercise:** Biceps Curl
   a. **Equipment:** Barbell (Fig. 5-70 and 5-71) or Universal Gym (Fig. 5-72 and 5-73)

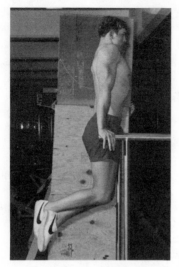

Figure 5-66. Starting
position for the **dip.**

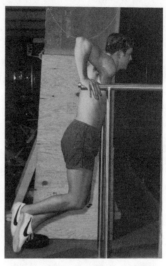

Figure 5-67. Execution of
the **dip.**

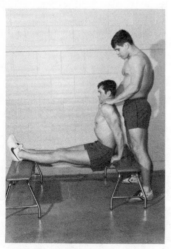

Figure 5-68. Starting
position for the **L-seat dip.**

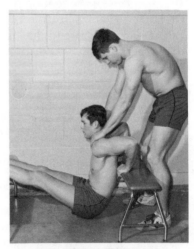

Figure 5-69. Execution
of the **L-seat dip.**

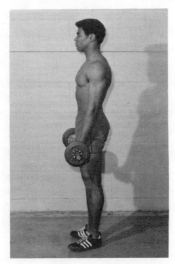

Figure 5-70. Starting position for the **biceps curl** with a barbell.

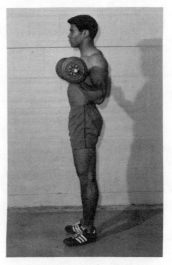

Figure 5-71. Execution of the **biceps curl** with a barbell.

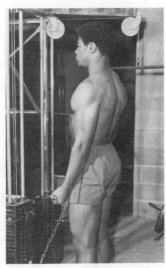

Figure 5-72. Starting position for the **biceps curl** on the Universal machine.

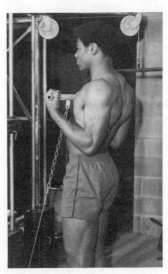

Figure 5-73. Execution of the **biceps curl** on the Universal machine.

b. **Muscles Used:** Biceps

c. **Prime Movers:** Biceps

d. **Starting Position:** Standing with the barbell hanging downward with the arms extended, an underhand grip should be used.

e. **Description:** Raise the barbell forward and upward until the biceps are fully contracted, pause momentarily and recover to the starting position.

f. **Breathing:** Inhale while raising the weight and exhale when recovering to the starting position.

g. **Spotting:** N/A

h. **Points to Emphasize:**

(1) Keep the elbows back throughout the entire exercise (this will keep resistance on the biceps in the contracted position); do not bring the elbows forward. (Fig. 5-74 incorrect technique)

(2) Keep the body perpendicular (do not lean backwards when raising the weight).

(3) Lower the weight slowly.

(4) When dumbbells are used the lifter should alternate the raising and lowering of the weight (Fig. 5-75 and 5-76).

(5) If dumbells are used, one dumbell should always be held in the contracted position.

6. **Exercise:** Wrist Curls (Fig. 5-77 and 5-78)

a. **Equipment:** Barbell, exercise bench

b. **Muscles Used:** Forearm flexors

c. **Prime Mover:** Forearm flexors

d. **Starting Position:** Seated with the forearms resting on the thighs, the back of the hands are against the knees; the fingers may be extended.

e. **Description:** Flex the wrists raising the barbell forward and upward, pause momentarily and recover to the starting position.

f. **Breathing:** Inhale while raising the weight and exhale when recovering to the starting position.

g. **Spotting:** N/A

h. **Points to Emphasize:**

(1) The forearm (Fig. 5-79) and elbow (Fig. 5-80) must remain in contact with the thigh to provide full range exercise.

(2) Lower the weight slowly.

7. **Exercise:** Reverse wrist curl (Fig. 5-81 and 5-82)

a. **Equipment:** Barbell

b. **Muscles Used:** Forearm extensors

c. **Prime Mover:** Forearm extensors

d. **Starting Position:** Seated with an overhand grip on the bar, the

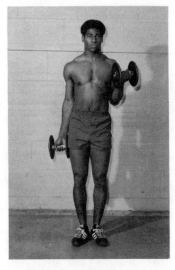

Figure 5-75. Starting position for the **biceps curl** with dumbells.

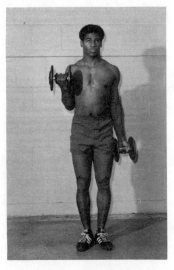

Figure 5-76. Execution of the **biceps curl** with dumbells.

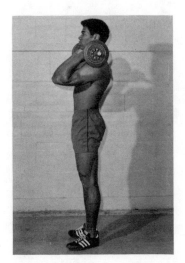

Figure 5-74. Incorrect technique for performing the **biceps curl.**

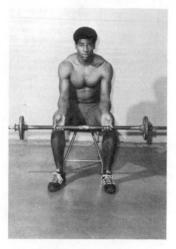

Figure 5-77. Starting position for the **wrist curl.**

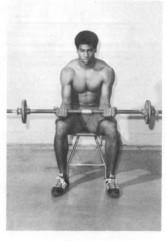

Figure 5-78. Execution of the **wrist curl.**

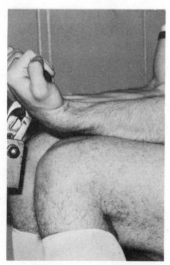

Figure 5-79. Correct position of the forearms during the **wrist curl.**

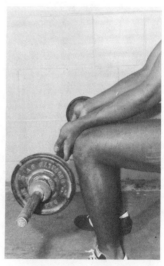

Figure 5-80. Incorrect position of the elbows during the **wrist curl.**

forearms and elbows are resting on the thighs; the palm of the hands are facing the knees.

e. **Description:** Extend the wrist forward and upward, pause momentarily and recover to the starting position.

f. **Breathing:** Inhale while raising the weight and exhale when recovering to the starting position.

g. **Spotting:** N/A

h. **Points to Emphasize:**

(1) Same as wrist curl.

(2) A reverse curl (Fig. 5-83 and 5-84) can be performed by performing a biceps curl with an overhand grip (this will place the emphasis on the forearm extensors also).

## EXERCISES FOR THE ABDOMINALS

1. **Exercise:** Situp (Fig. 5-85 and 5-86)

a. **Equipment:** Situp board, exercise bench or floor, & pad to elevate the hips.

b. **Muscles Used:** Hip flexors, quadriceps, abdominals

c. **Prime Mover:** Abdominals

d. **Starting Position:** Seated on a pad resting on the floor with the feet close to the buttocks, knees together, hands interlocked behind the head, with the buttocks elevated, the upperbody leaning slightly backwards (so that the abdominals are contracted).

e. **Description:** Lower the body to a position where the upper back is not quite touching the floor, pause momentarily and recover to the starting position.

f. **Breathing:** Inhale while lowering the upper body and exhale when recovering to the starting position.

g. **Spotting:** Hold the lifter's feet if necessary. When performing negative only situps you should assist the lifter in recovering to the starting position.

h. **Points to Emphasize:**

(1) The hips should be elevated to prevent the back from touching the floor; this will prevent the abdominals from momentarily recovering during each repetition.

(2) When raising the upper body do not come to a position where the torso is perpendicular to the floor. This will allow the abdominals to relax and recover momentarily (you should raise the upper body as far as possible while maintaining some tension on the abdominals).

(3) Allow the **muscles** to raise the body and not momentum (raise the body slowly while keeping the elbows stationary (4 seconds to raise the body).

(4) It should take approximately 6-8 seconds to lower the body.

(5) Weight can be added by placing a barbell plate on the chest

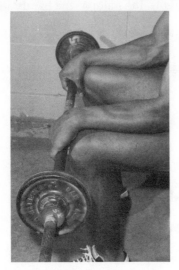

Figure 5-81. Starting position for the **reverse wrist curl**.

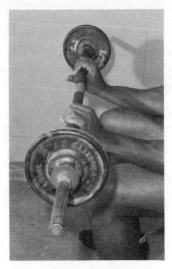

Figure 5-82. Execution of the **reverse wrist curl.**

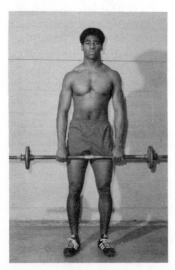

Figure 5-83. Starting position for the **reverse wrist curl** performed by a biceps curl with an overhand grip.

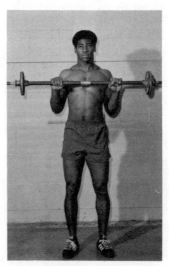

Figure 5-84. Execution of the **reverse wrist curl** performed by a biceps curl with an overhand grip.

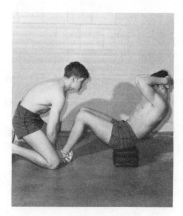

Figure 5-85. Starting
position for the **situp**.

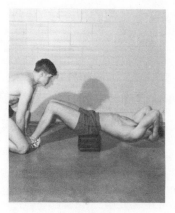

Figure 5-86. Execution
of the **situp**.

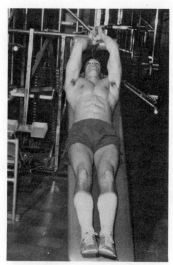

Figure 5-87. Starting
position for the **leg raise**.

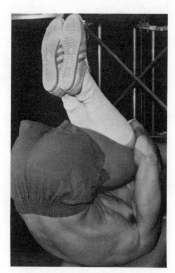

Figure 5-88. Execution
of the **leg raise**.

(not behind the head, places more stress on lower back) or a spotter may provide additional resistance by pulling the lifter downward while he lowers his torso.

(6) The higher the hips are elevated the greater the difficulty and the greater the stress on the lower back. Be cautious. (Adapt to the elevation of the hips slowly, support the lower back if necessary).

2. **Exercise:** Leg Raise (Fig. 5-87 and 5-88)
   a. **Equipment:** Abdominal or incline board
   b. **Muscles Used:** Abdominals, hip flexors
   c. **Prime Mover:** Abdominals
   d. **Starting Position:** Lying on the back on an incline board, grasp the bench to stabilize the body. The legs are extended with the heels just barely off the abdominal board.
   e. **Description:** Bend the legs drawing the heels toward the buttocks and then draw the knees up toward the forehead, pause momentarily and recover to the starting position.
   f. **Breathing:** Inhale while raising the legs and exhale when recovering to the starting position.
   g. **Spotting:** To increase the intensity of the exercise a spotter can apply resistance to the legs.
   h. **Points to Emphasize:**
   
   (1) As the angle of the incline board increases, so will the difficulty of the exercise.
   
   (2) The legs may be kept straight throughout the entire exercise to increase the difficulty.
   
   (3) You may bend the legs to raise them and straighten them when lowering (you can lower more weight than you can raise).
   
   (4) Weights may be attached to the feet to increase the difficulty of the exercise.
   
   (5) Do not hang from a chin bar to perform the exercise (once you have developed a sufficient level of abdominal strength your grip will fail before your abdominals).
   
   (6) The speed of movement should be very slow to allow the abdominals and not momentum to perform the work.
   
   (7) Adjust the angle of the board so that you are capable of performing 8-12 properly executed repetitions (quality not quantity).

## EXERCISES FOR THE NECK

1. **Exercise:** Neck Curl (Fig. 5-89 and 5-90)
   a. **Equipment:** Exercise bench
   b. **Muscles Used:** Flexors

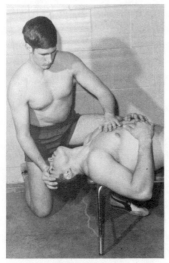

Figure 5-89. Starting position for the **neck curl** using an exercise bench.

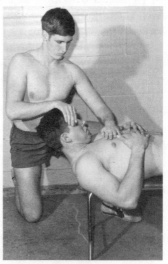

Figure 5-90. Execution of the **neck curl** using an exercise bench.

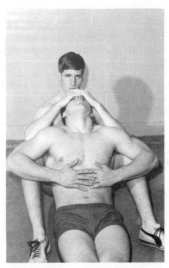

Figure 5-91. Starting position for the **neck curl** without an exercise bench.

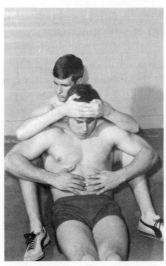

Figure 5-92. Execution of the **neck curl** without an exercise bench.

c. **Prime Movers:** Flexors

d. **Starting Position:** Lying on the back on an exercise bench, only the head should be hanging over the end of the bench; the top of the head should be parallel with the floor, arms folded across the chest, feet flat on the floor, neck muscles relaxed.

e. **Description:** Flexing only the neck muscles raise the head forward and upward so that the chin is resting on the chest; "pause momentarily" and recover to the starting position.

f. **Breathing:** Inhale while raising the head and exhale when recovering to the starting position.

g. **Spotting:** Place your hand on the lifter's forehead and apply only as much pressure as is needed to permit the lifter to perform 8-12 properly executed repetitions.

h. **Points to Emphasize:**

(1) Never exercise the neck muscles before a practice in which head contact and collisions will occur, (muscles will be weaker and more susceptible to injury), stretch before and exercise after practice.

(2) Never perform an isometric exercise for the neck muscles (flexibility is reduced and strength is only gained at one fixed point).

(3) Any neck exercise **must** be performed **slowly** without any jerky movements.

(4) Spotting must be emphasized.

(a) Practice spotting techniques thoroughly before performing the exercise all out.

(b) Request that the lifter perform a few practice repetitions so that you may ensure he is performing the exercise properly.

(c) You must adjust the amount of pressure applied to accommodate for the strength curve of the neck flexors (more pressure should be applied when the lifter is lowering the head than when he is raising it).

(d) The lifter should pause momentarily when the neck is completely flexed (chin on chest) and extended (top of the head parallel to the floor).

(e) The spotter should apply **very little** pressure when the neck is **approaching the extended position** (the tendency of the lifter will be to tense up at this position which will prevent full range exercise and stretching).

(f) Constant interaction between spotter and lifter is necessary to provide maximum efficiency.

(g) The lifter should only move the head (do not raise the back off the bench).

(h) Can be performed without an exercise bench (Fig. 5-91 and 5-92).

2. **Exercise:** Neck Extension (Fig. 5-93 and 5-94)

a. **Equipment:** Exercise bench

b. **Muscles Used:** Neck extensors

c. **Prime Movers:** Neck extensors

d. **Starting Position:** Lay face down on an exercise bench with the head hanging over the edge of the bench, the head should be flexed so that the chin is touching the chest. The hands should be resting behind the back, neck muscles relaxed.

e. **Description:** Raise the head forward and upward until the head is fully extended, pause momentarily and recover to the starting position.

f. **Breathing:** Inhale while raising the weight and exhale when lowering the weight.

g. **Spotting:** Place a hand on the back of the lifter's head and apply as much resistance as is needed so that the lifter can only perform 8-12 properly executed repetitions.

h. **Points to Emphasize:**

(1) Same as the neck curl exercise.

(2) The head should be far enough off the exercise bench so that the chin will not make contact with the bench.

(3) Do not lift the chest off the bench (only move the head).

(4) The neck extension exercise can be performed with the lifter assuming a position on his hands and knees (Fig. 5-95 and 5-96).

3. **Exercise:** Lateral Neck Flexion (Fig. 5-96 and 5-97)

a. **Equipment:** Exercise bench

b. **Muscles Used:** Lateral flexors

c. **Prime Mover:** Lateral flexors

d. **Starting Position:** Lying on the back on an exercise bench, the head may be extended over the edge of the bench; the back of the head should be parallel to the floor; the head should be in a flexed position to one side.

e. **Description:** Move the head sideward moving the lateral flexors through their full range of motion, pause momentarily and recover.

f. **Breathing:** Normal cadence

g. **Spotting:** Place one hand on the right side of the lifter's head and apply as much pressure as is needed so that the lifter is only capable of performing 8-12 properly executed reps, then place your hand on the left side of the lifter's head and again have the lifter perform 8-12 properly executed reps.

h. **Points to Emphasize:**

(1) Same as the neck curl and neck extension exercise.*

(2) Gradually decrease the resistance being applied when the lifter approaches the extended position (allow him to stretch the muscles). If

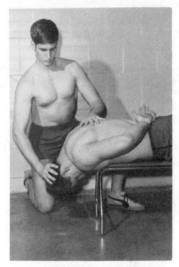

Figure 5-93. Starting position for the **neck extension** using an exercise bench.

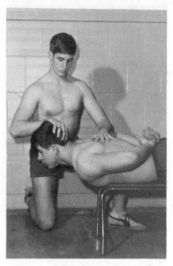

Figure 5-94. Execution of the **neck extension** using an exercise bench.

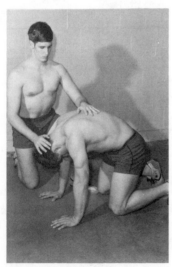

Figure 5-95. Starting position for the **neck extension** on the hands and knees.

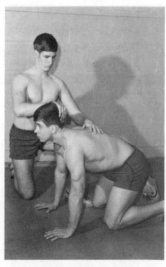

Figure 5-96. Execution of the **neck extension** on the hands and knees.

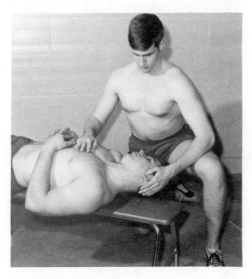

Figure 5-97. Starting position for the **lateral neck flexion**.

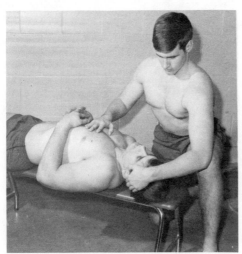

Figure 5-98. Execution of the **lateral neck flexion**.

too much resistance is applied he will tighten up and not go through the full range of movement.

(3) The shoulders should remain stationary throughout the entire exercise.

(4) The lifter may be in the seated position to perform the lateral neck flexion exercise.

*Credit for all photographs used in this chapter should be given to "U.S. Army Photographs".

# CHAPTER 6
## Nautilus Training

Daniel P. Riley
Director of Strength Training

Nautilus exercises

Nautilus training is a type of training which utilizes Nautilus weight training machines as the equipment for the exercise. Developed by Arthur Jones, these machines have revolutionized many of the concepts and practices of "muscular development" training. The complete line of Nautilus equipment is gradually increasing every year, currently numbering more than 20 separate machines. Each machine is designed to provide for the "seven requirements" of exercise: (1) full-range resistance; (2) direct resistance; (3) balanced resistance; (4) omni-directional resistance; (5) automatically-variable resistance; (6) rotary-form resistance; and (7) Negative-work potential.

The format for this chapter is similar to that used for Chapter 5. For each exercise, the following information is presented: the required equipment, the muscles effected, the starting position for the exercise, a description of how to perform the exercise, breathing instructions, spotting hints, and points to emphasize.

## NAUTILUS EXERCISES
### SUPER HIP AND BACK

**Exercise:** Super Hip and Back
**Equipment:** Super Geared Hip and Back Machine.
**Muscles Used:** Buttocks, lower back muscles.
**Starting Position:** Lying on the back on the hip and back machine with the shoulders in contact with the shoulder pads on the sliding carriage, the axis of rotation of the hips should be aligned with the center of the nautilus cam, knees should be together and remain together throughout the exercise, grasp the pair of stationary handles on the front of the machine with the fingers extended in joint (this will force the athlete to push with the hands keeping the shoulders in contact with the pads instead of pulling with the hands when the weight is being lowered).
**Description:** Extend from the hip forward and downward until the buttocks are fully contracted (the body should be in an arched position), pause momentarily and recover to the starting position.
**Breathing:** Inhale when recovering to the starting position and exhale while extending the legs.

**Spotting:** To save time, the lifter can hold back on the left handle on the sliding carriage and the spotter can push the lifter into the proper starting position.

**To Assume the Starting Position:**

    a. Secure the seatbelt across the two bony parts of the hips so that in the contracted position, the back is arched slightly.

    b. Grasp the two movable handles on the sliding carriage.

    c. Pull the left handle back and hold it back while cranking the right handle back and forth until the proper starting position is assumed.

**Points to Emphasize:**

    1. The shorter athlete may have to add additional pads to the existing shoulder pads on the sliding carriage (this will allow the shoulders to remain in contact with the shoulder pads throughout the entire range of movement).

    2. Getting out of the machine upon completion of the exercise.

        a. Push both handles on the sliding carriage forward and hold them there.

    3. A standard barbell plate (5, 10, or 20 pounds) can be pinned to the weight stack of the machine to provide for a smaller increase in weights (a 25 pound increase will be too much of an increment to allow proper execution and the desired number of repetitions.

**Advantages:** The buttocks are the prime mover in most movements responsible for the success of an athlete. However, with conventional equipment, the athlete is unable to isolate the buttocks. An exercise similar to the squat or leg press must be performed to involve the buttocks which is the largest and strongest muscle group in the body. Unfortunately, when performing these exercises, the smaller and weaker muscles of the legs fail first. It is impossible to exercise the buttocks to the point of failure without the Nautilus hip and back machine.


## DUO-POLY HIP AND BACK

**Exercise:** Duo-Poly Hip and Back.

**Equipment:** Duo-Poly Hip and Back Machine.

**Muscles Used:** Buttocks, lower back.

**Starting Position:** Lying on the back on the hip and back machine with the axis of rotation of the hips aligned with the axis of rotation of the Nautilus cam, grasp the stationary handles with the hands (fingers extended in joint) (push don't pull), seatbelt on the duo poly should be tightly across the bony parts of the hips (not the stomach). Both legs should be extended from the hips with the toes pointed and legs straight (do not bend the legs attempting to touch the floor with the feet).

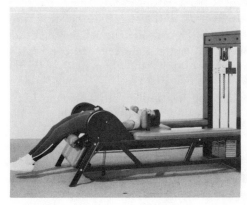

Execution of the Nautilus **Super Hip & Back.**

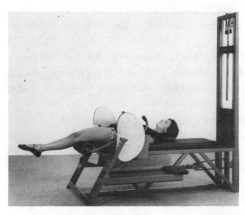

Starting position for the Nautilus **Duo-Poly Hip & Back.**

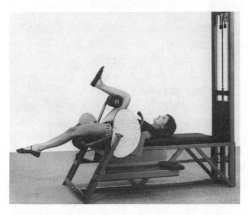

Execution of the Nautilus **Duo-Poly Hip & Back.**

**Description:** The right leg will remain stationary in the contracted position while the left leg moves backwards to the stretched position (pre-stretch) and then recover to the starting position. The left leg will then remain in the contracted position while the right leg is moved backwards to the stretched position (pre-stretch) and then recover to the starting position.

**Breathing:** Exhale while extending the leg and inhale when the leg is moved backwards.

**Points to Emphasize:**

1. Arms should remain extended throughout the entire exercise (do not pull with the hands as the leg is being extended).

2. The leg that remains extended should not move at all while the other leg is being exercised.

a. If the leg remaining in the extended position moves at any time while raising or lowering the weight with the leg being exercised, the weight is too heavy or you are coming back too far with the leg being exercised.

**Advantages:** The duo poly hip and back machine isolates the same muscles as the super geared hip and back while the exercising principle varies slightly. By keeping one leg in the contracted position it can minimize cheating. Also, each leg is exercised separately preventing the dominant leg from performing most of the work.


## LEG EXTENSION

**Exercise:** Leg Extension.

**Equipment:** Leg Extension Machine.

**Muscles Used:** Knee Extensors.

**Prime Mover:** Quadriceps.

**Starting Position:** Sitting on the extension machine with the top of the feet hooked under the pads on the moment arm, the back of the knee should be in contact with the front edge of the padded seat, leaning back with the hands cupped grasping the hand grips on the side of the machine, head and shoulders against the seat back.

**Description:** Extend the legs until they are completely extended, pause momentarily in the contracted position and recover to the starting position (do not let the weight plates being lifted return to the weight stack — this will allow the muscles to momentarily recover).

**Breathing:** Inhale while lowering the weight and exhale when raising the weight.

**Points to Emphasize:**

1. The same seat adjustment should be used each time the exercise is performed.

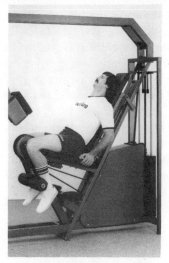

Starting position for the
Nautilus **Leg Extension**

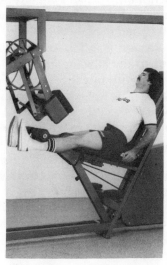

Execution of the Nautilus
**Leg Extension**

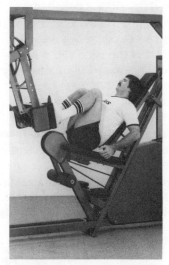

Starting position for the
Nautilus **Leg Press**

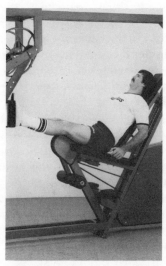

Execution of the Nautilus
**Leg Press**

2. If the lifter cannot pause momentarily in the legs extended position, the weight is too heavy or the athlete has reached the point of failure.

3. Do not lean forward while lowering the weight (this will prevent the muscle from being stretched).

4. Do not raise the buttocks off the padded seat, especially when lowering the weight (this will also prevent the muscle from being stretched).

5. Do not squeeze the hand grips used to keep the buttocks in contact with the seat (cup the hands).

6. To move the seat backwards simply pull the rear hand grip on the right side of the seat—this will release the locking mechanism and allow the seat to move freely.

7. If the compound leg machine is used, the athlete should initiate the leg press exercise immediately upon completion of the leg extension exercise.


## LEG PRESS

**Exercise:** Leg Press.

**Equipment:** Compound Leg Machine.

**Muscles Used:** Major muscles of the legs and buttocks.

**Prime Movers:** Buttocks, Quadriceps.

**Starting Position:** Seated with the feet on the leg press pedals, foot pad should be lowered to the down position for the leg press exercise, the arch of the feet should be placed on the **center** of the leg press pedals (when the toes are placed on the lower part of the pedals, the mechanical advantage is better but undue stress will be placed upon the knees), the seat should be adjusted so that legs form a 90° angle or less (full range exercise).

**Description:** Extend the legs until they are almost extended (do not allow the legs to "lockout"—this will allow the muscles to recover), and then return to the starting position without allowing the weight plates being lifted to touch the weight stack not being lifted.

**Spotting:** The exercise is started in a position where there is a distinct mechanical disadvantage—the spotter should therefore assist the lifter to initiate the first repetition by pushing with his hands on the foot pedals of the leg press machine.

**Points to Emphasize:**

1. The seat should be in the same position each time the exercise is performed.

2. If headaches occur during the exercise, observe the following:

    a. Do not squeeze the hands while grasping the hand grips (cup

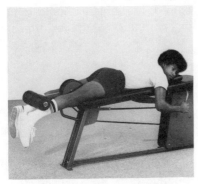

Starting position for the
Nautilus **Leg Curl.**

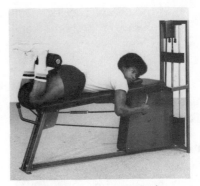

Execution of the Nautilus
**Leg Curl.**

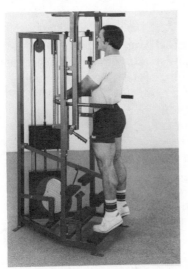

Execution of the **Heel Raise**
on the Nautilus Multi-
Exercise Machine.

the hands).

    b. Do not hold the breath.

    c. Move the seat back a notch each workout until headaches disappear.

    3. The buttocks should remain in contact with the seat throughout the exercise.

    4. If the compound leg machine is used, the athlete should initiate the leg press exercise immediately upon completion of the leg extension exercise.

## LEG CURL

**Exercise:** Leg Curl.

**Equipment:** Leg Curl Machine.

**Muscles Used:** Knee flexors.

**Prime Mover:** Hamstrings.

**Starting Position:** Lying face down on the leg curl machine with the heels hooked under the pads on the moment arm, the kneecap should be just off the edge of the pad for comfort and efficiency, ankles flexed.

**Description:** Flex the lower legs pulling them upward and forward until the legs are at least perpendicular to the floor, pause momentarily and recover to the starting position, ankles should remain flexed throughout the exercise.

**Breathing:** Inhale while raising the weight and exhale when recovering to the starting position.

**Points to Emphasize:**

    1. A belt or strap can be used to secure the hips to the pad.

    2. When lowering the weight, the hips should remain in contact with the pad to provide for maximum stretching of the muscles involved.

## HEEL RAISE

**Exercise:** Heel Raise.

**Equipment:** Multi-Exercise Machine.

**Muscles Used:** Foot extensors.

**Prime Mover:** Calves.

**Starting Position:** Standing on the first step of the multi-exercise machine leaning forward so that the calves are in the stretched position, the body should be straight, do not bend at the waist, ankles are relaxed with the heels lower than the toes to provide for maximum stretching, the waist belt secured to the weight stack can be attached to the waist to increase the resistance.

**Description:** Raise the heel upward until the calves have contracted completely, pause momentarily and recover to the starting position.

**Points to Emphasize:**

1. While leaning forward, do not use the arms to push downward on the machine, this would assist the calves in raising the weight.

2. As the lifter fatigues, there will be a tendency to increase the speed of movement while raising the weight.

3. Do not lean back while lowering the heels, this will prevent maximum stretching of the calves.

## SIDE LATERAL RAISE

**Exercise:** Side Lateral Raise (primary movement).

**Equipment:** Nautilus Double Shoulder Machine.

**Prime Mover:** Deltoids.

**Starting Position:** Seated with the axis of rotation of the shoulders aligned with the axis of rotation of the Nautilus cam, grasp the hand grips used for the side lateral raise placing the back of the wrists up against the pads available, pull back on the hand grips as far as possible, the elbows should be parallel with the hands, shoulders and lower back resting against seat back.

**Description:** Raise the hands and arms upward leading with the elbows (do not drop the elbows and lead with the hands), continue to raise the arms until the upperarm makes contact with the handles used for the seated press exercise, pause momentarily and recover to the starting position.

**Breathing:** Inhale while raising the weight and exhale when recovering to the starting position.

**Points to Emphasize:**

1. Lead with the elbows and not the hands.

2. The deltoids will have contracted when the elbows are just above parallel to the floor (to raise the weight higher could detract from the efficiency of the exercise.

3. A conscious effort must be made throughout the exercise to pull back with the hands and not push forward.

4. If the feet are resting on the floor, do not use the legs to assist in raising the weight by standing up (athletes with large legs may find difficulty keeping the legs on the seat).

5. The same seat setting will be used for the seated press and side lateral raise exercise.

6. Upon completion of the side lateral raise exercise the spotter should make a weight adjustment if necessary so that the lifter can immediately initiate the secondary movement, the seated press.

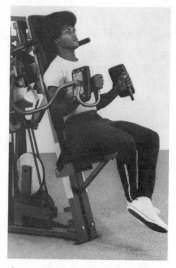

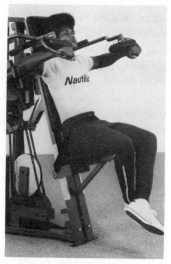

Starting position for the **Side Lateral Raise** on the Nautilus Double Shoulder Machine

Execution of the **Side Lateral Raise** on the Nautilus Double Shoulder Machine

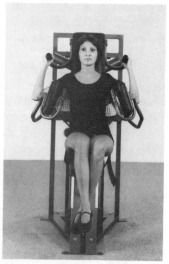

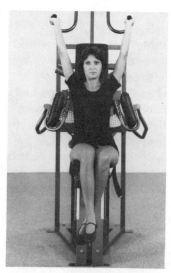

Starting position for the **Seated Press** on the Nautilus Double Shoulder Machine

Execution of the **Seated Press** on the Nautilus Double Shoulder Machine

## SEATED PRESS

**Exercise:** Seated Press (secondary movement)
**Equipment:** Double Shoulder Machine.
**Muscles Used:** Deltoids, triceps.
**Prime Mover:** Deltoids.
**Starting Position:** Seated with the hands grasping the hand grips used for the seated press exercise, body in the same position otherwise.
**Description:** Extend the arms upward so that the arms become momentarily extended and recover to the starting position.
**Breathing:** Inhale while lowering the weight and exhale when raising the weight.
**Points to Emphasize:**

1. The lifter should initiate the seated press exercise as quickly as possible upon completion of the side lateral raise exercise.

   a. A weight adjustment may be necessary—depending upon Ihe individual and his length of arms, the athlete may use more weight on either of the exercises.

2. If the legs are straddling the seat and the feet are resting on the floor, do not use the legs to raise the weight.

3. Arching the back will place undue stress on the lower back (the athlete is trying to recruit the pectorals to assist).

4. Do not rest in the arms extended position.


## BENT ARM FLY

**Exercise:** Bent Arm Fly (primary movement).
**Equipment:** Double Chest Machine.
**Prime Mover:** Pectorals.
**Starting Position:** Seated with the axis of rotation of the shoulders aligned with the overhead Nautilus cams (when the elbows are together) forearms should be placed behind the pads used to perform the exercise, the thumbs are hooked under the top handgrips (the handgrips should meet the junction of the thumb and index finger).
**Description:** Move the forearms forward until the pectorals are fully contracted, pause momentarily, and recover to the starting position.
**Spotting:** If there is a need to adjust the weight for the decline press, the spotter should make the adjustment immediately upon completion of the bent arm fly so that the lifter can initiate the secondary movement as quickly as possible.
**Points to Emphasize:**

1. If proper alignment is attained in the starting position, the elbows will be a few inches higher than the axis of rotation of the shoulders.

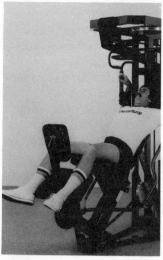

Starting position for the **Bent Arm Fly** on the Nautilus Double Chest Machine

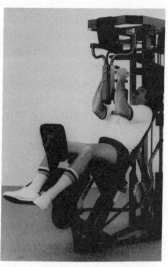

Execution of the **Bent Arm Fly** on the Nautilus Double Chest Machine

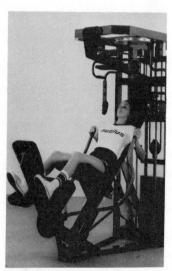

Starting position for the **Decline Press** on the Nautilus Double Chest Machine

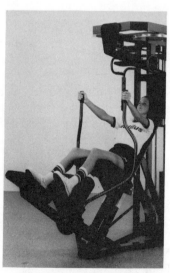

Execution of the **Decline Press** on the Nautilus Double Chest Machine

2. Do not grasp the hand grips making a fist because there will then be a tendency to push with the hands and not the forearms, which in turn would decrease the efficiency of the exercise.

3. The same seat adjustment will be used to perform both exercises on this machine.

4. Do not lean forward with the head and torso when raising the weight.

5. The seat belt can be secured to prevent unnecessary movement.

## DECLINE PRESS

**Exercise:** Decline Press (secondary movement).
**Equipment:** Double Chest Machine.
**Muscles Used:** Pectorals, Deltoids, Triceps.
**Prime Mover:** Pectorals.
**Starting Position:** Seated with the hands grasping the hand grips on the decline press, the arms should be extended, the same seat adjustment should be used that was used for the bent arm fly exercise.
**Assume the Starting Position:**

a. Secure seat belt.

b. Place the feet on the foot pedal and extend the legs simultaneously grasping the hand grips and extending the arms to the arms extended position.

**Description:** Lower the weight so that the pectorals are fully stretched and recover to the starting position.
**Breathing:** Inhale while lowering the weight and exhale when recovering to the starting position.
**Points to Emphasize:**

1. Upon completion of the exercise place the feet on the foot pad and extend the legs until the hands can be removed from the hand grips, the weight can then be returned to the weight stack by using the legs and not the arms.

2. Do not remain in the arms extended position upon completion of each repetition (this will allow the muscles to momentarily recover to the starting position).

## PULLOVER

**Exercise:** Pullover.
**Equipment:** Nautilus Pullover Machine.
**Prime Mover:** Latissimus Dorsi.
**Starting Position:** Seated with the axis of rotation of the shoulders approximately 3 inches below the axis of rotation of the Nautilus cams,

elbows placed on the pads available, the side of the hands are placed on the pullover bar, the pullover bar should be resting against the waist with the torso perpendicular to the floor, seat belt secured.

**To Assume the Starting Position:**

1. Place the feet on the foot pedal available and extend the legs.
2. Place the elbows on the elbow pads and the side of the hands (in a karate chop manner) on the pullover bar.
3. Driving with the elbows, bring the pullover bar to a position where it is resting against the waist.
4. Remove the feet from the foot pedals allowing the footlever to recover to its original position.

**Description:** Lower the weight allowing the pullover bar to move upward and backward through the lifter's full range of movement allowing the shoulder girdle and latissimus dorsi to be fully stretched and recover to the starting position.

**Breathing:** Inhale while lowering the weight and exhale when recovering to the starting position.

**Points to Emphasize:**

1. Do not lean forward when raising or lowering the weight.
2. The head and shoulders should remain stationary throughout the entire exercise.
3. A conscious effort must be made to drive with the elbows and not pull with the hands.
4. Unless hand grips are available, the lifter should maintain contact with the pullover bar with the side of the hand (do not grasp the bar wrapping the fingers around the bar).
5. If the lifter cannot pause momentarily in the starting position, the weight is too heavy or the athlete has reached the point of failure.
6. Upon completion of the exercise place the feet on the foot lever and extend the legs until there is no resistance being applied to the elbows, remove the arms and return the weight to the weight stack by using the legs.

## DUO-POLY PULLOVER

**Exercise:** Duo-Poly Pullover.

**Equipment:** Duo-Poly Pullover.

**Prime Mover:** Latissimus Dorsi.

**Starting Position:** Seated with the seat belt secured, the seat should be adjusted so that the axis of rotation of the shoulders are aligned with the axis of the Nautilus cams when the latissimus is in the stretched position, both movement arms should be in the midrange position, the torso and head erect, the fingers extended with the side of the hand placed on

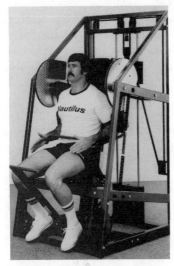

Starting position for the Nautilus **Pullover**

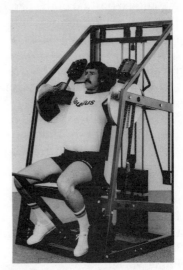

Execution of the Nautilus **Pullover**

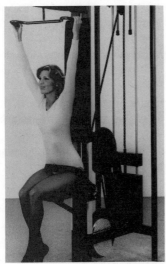

Starting position for the **Lat Pulldown** on the Nautilus Torso Arm Machine

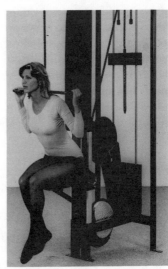

Execution of the **Lat Pulldown** on the Nautilus Torso Arm Machine

the curved portion of the bar, elbows placed on pads available.

**Description:** Rotate one arm back as far as possible to the stretched position (keeping the other arm in the contracted position) and recover to the starting position, repeat with the other arm.

**Breathing:** Inhale as the weight is being lowered and exhale when recovering to the starting position.

**Points to Emphasize:**

1. Do not move the head or torso.

2. Insure that the arm remaining in the contracted position does not move while the other arm is being exercised.

## LAT PULLDOWN

**Exercise:** Lat Pulldown.

**Equipment:** Nautilus Torso Arm Machine.

**Muscles Used:** Latissimus Dorsi, Biceps, Posterior Deltoids.

**Prime Mover:** Latissimus Dorsi.

**Starting Position:** Seated on the torso arm machine with the seat belt secured, arms extended with the hands grasping the two hand grips (with the palms facing each other), the seat should be low enough so that the latissimus dorsi are fully stretched.

**Spotting:** The spotter should pull the bar downward so that the lifter can grasp the handles (in the starting position the seat should be low enough so that the lifter cannot quite reach the hand grips on the torso arm bar).

**Description:** Pull the torso arm bar downward to a position behind the neck, pause momentarily and recover to the starting position.

**Breathing:** Inhale while pulling the bar downward and exhale when recovering to the starting position.

**Points to Emphasize:**

1. If a combination pullover torso arm machine is being used, the lifter upon completion of the pullover exercise should immediately initiate the torso arm exercise.

2. The lifter should then drive the elbows downward and backward until the torso arm bar touches the chest, pause momentarily, and recover to the starting position.

3. The athlete should drive with the elbows instead of pulling with the biceps.

4. The seat should be lowered to provide maximum stretching.

## TRICEPS EXTENSION

**Exercise:** Triceps Extension.

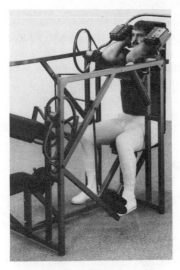

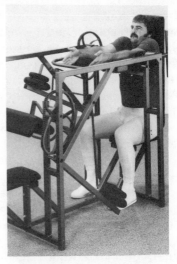

Starting position for the **Triceps Extension** on the Nautilus Biceps-Triceps Machine

Execution of the **Triceps Extension** on the Nautilus Biceps-Triceps Machine

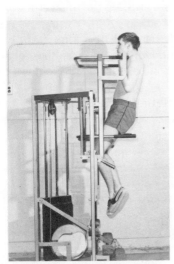

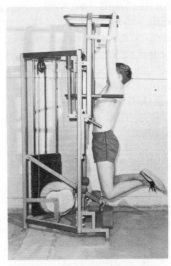

Starting position for the **Chinup** on the Nautilus Multi-Exercise Machine

Execution of the **Chinup** on the Nautilus Multi-Exercise Machine

**Equipment:** Nautilus Biceps-Triceps Machine.
**Prime Mover:** Triceps.
**Starting Position:** Seated with the elbows resting on the pad available, the side of the hands (in a karate chop manner) should be placed against the pads on the extension bar, the triceps are in the stretched position.
**Description:** Extend the arms forward and downward until the arms are extended, pause momentarily, and recover to the starting position.
**Breathing:** Inhale while recovering to the starting position and exhale when extending the arms.
**Points to Emphasize:**

1. Every attempt should be made to maintain contact with the elbows and the pad they rest upon.

2. Pads may be added to the seat to elevate the lifter and place him into the proper lifting position (the arms should be parallel with the floor when the arms are fully extended).

3. The lifter should maintain contact with the extension pads and the **side** of the hands, while extending the arms there is a tendency to rotate the hands pushing with palms of the hands and not the sides.


## CHINUP

**Exercise:** Chinup.
**Equipment:** Nautilus Multi-Exercise Machine.
**Muscles Used:** Latissimus Dorsi, Biceps.
**Prime Mover:** Latissimus Dorsi.
**Starting Position:** Hanging from the chin bar with the arms fully extended, a closer than shoulder width and underhand grip should be used, the knees should be flexed to prevent the feet from touching the floor.
**Description:** Raise the chin to the bar by flexing the arms until they are fully contracted, pause momentarily and recover to the starting position.
**Breathing:** Inhale while raising the bodyweight and exhale when recovering to the starting position.
**Points to Emphasize:**

1. Once 12 properly executed repetitions can be performed, the lifter can secure the waist strap to the movement arm which is attached to the weight stack of the Multi-Exercise machine.

    a. The waist strap can then be placed around the lifter's waist which will increase the resistance of the exercise.

2. Reemphasize to the athletes that they are trying to develop strength and not demonstrate it (it is not how many chinups you perform that counts, it is how you perform them) the speed of movement while raising and lowering the weight should be controlled.

3. Negative chinups can and should be performed every other workout.

    a. More resistance will be needed to perform negative chinups.

    b. Lower the bodyweight slowly (at least 8 seconds per repetition).

    c. Upon completion of each repetition, the lifter must recover to the starting position as quickly as possible to initiate the next repetition (do not allow the muscles to momentarily recover by taking too much time to initiate the next repetition).

## DIPS

**Exercise:** Dips.

**Equipment:** Nautilus Multi-Exercise Machine.

**Muscles Used:** Pectorals, Deltoids, Triceps.

**Starting Position:** Mounted on the dip bars with the arms extended, knees should be bent.

**Description:** Bend the arms lowering the body, stretching the muscles involved as much as possible, and recover to the starting position.

**Breathing:** Inhale while lowering the body and exhale when recovering to the starting position.

**Points to Emphasize:**

1. Once 12 properly executed repetitions can be performed, the athlete can attach additional weight to the body.

2. The body should be lowered as far as possible to provide maximum stretching and full range exercise.

3. Negative only dips can and should be performed every other workout.

    a. More resistance will be needed to perform negative dips.

    b. Lower the bodyweight slowly (at least 8 seconds to lower the bodyweight).

    c. Upon completion of each repetition, the lifter must recover to the starting position as quickly as possible to initiate the next repetition (do not allow the muscles to momentarily recover by taking too much time to initiate the next repetition).

## SHOULDER SHRUGS

**Exercise:** Shoulder Shrugs.

**Equipment:** Nautilus Shrug Machine.

**Prime Mover:** Trapezius.

**Starting Position:** Seated on the shrug machine with the forearms placed between the upper and lower pads available, the palms are facing skyward, the arms must be pushed forward so that the biceps are in contact

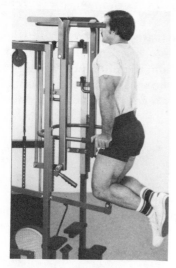

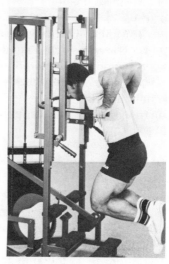

Starting position for the **Dip** on the Nautilus Multi-Exercise Machine

Execution of the **Dip** on the Nautilus Multi-Exercise Machine

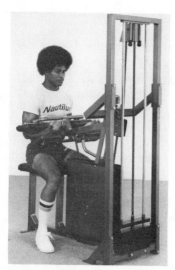

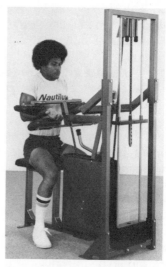

Starting position for the **Shoulder Shrug** on the Nautilus Shrug Machine

Execution of the **Shoulder Shrug** on the Nautilus Shrug Machine with the side of the upper pads, the back of the hands should be pushing downward against the lower pads, the torso erect, the weight plates being lifted should not be touching the weight stack (this will provide for maximum stretching and full range exercise).

**Description:** Elevate the shoulder girdle as high as possible (using only the trapezius), pause momentarily and recover to the starting position.

**Breathing:** Inhale while raising the weight and exhale when recovering to the starting position.

**Points to Emphasize:**

1. Do not lean backwards while raising the weight.

2. Do not use the arms to assist in raising the weight.

3. Sit up straight while lowering the weight (do not lean forward, this will decrease the range of movement and prevent maximum stretching).

4. Push downward with the back of the hands, the fingers should be extended (do not make a fist).

5. The biceps should remain in contact with the sides of the upper two pads throughout the exercise.

6. Shoulder shrugs can be performed on the multi-exercise machine by attaching the shrug handle to the movement arm.

**Advantages:** The Nautilus shrug machine was designed to isolate and strengthen the trapezius, a very large and strong muscle of the neck and upperback. The Nautilus cam varies the resistance in such a way that very little weight is needed to elicit an all out effort. The resistance is directly applied to the forearms which eliminates the use of the hands gripping a barbell. The trapezius is a much larger and stronger muscle than the gripping muscles of the forearms. Consequently, when using a barbell you are limited to a resistance which the weaker muscles of the forearms are capable of holding during the exercise. Therefore, the trapezius muscle is never exercised to the point of failure.

## NECK EXTENSION

**Exercise:** Neck Extension.

**Equipment:** 4-way Neck Machine.

**Prime Mover:** Neck Extensors.

**Starting Position:** Seated with the back of the head resting against the pads available, the torso erect, the head looking downward placing the neck muscles in the stretched position (the weight plates being lifted should not touch the remaining weight stack) the back of the head and neck should be in contact with the pads (not just the top of the head), the seat adjustment should be low enough so that the extensors can be fully contracted while looking skyward (if the seat is too high, the bottom of the two pads will be touching the trapezius while extending

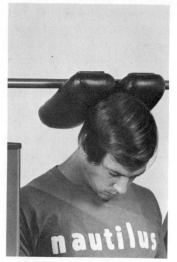

Starting position for the **Neck Extension** on the Nautilus 4-Way Neck Machine

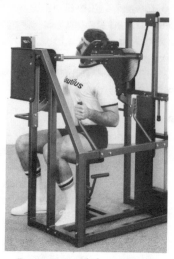

Execution of the **Lateral Neck Flexion** on the Nautilus 4-Way Neck Machine

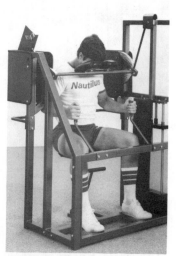

Starting position for the **Neck Flexion** on the Nautilus 4-Way Neck Machine

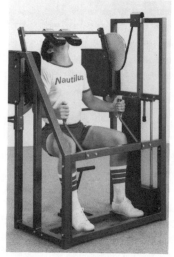

Execution of the **Neck Flexion** on the Nautilus 4-Way Neck Machine

the head backwards which will prevent full range exercise).

**Description:** Extend the head backwards looking skyward, pause momentarily and recover to the starting position.

**Breathing:** Inhale while extending the head backwards and exhale when recovering to the starting position.

**Points to Emphasize:**

1. All movements should be controlled, performed slowly.

2. Do not lean forward when the weight is being lowered (sit erect throughout the exercise).

3. Do not lean backwards when raising the weight (allow the muscles to raise the weight and not the weight of the body leaning backwards).

## NECK FLEXION

**Exercise:** Neck Flexion.

**Equipment:** 4-Way Neck Machine.

**Prime Mover:** Neck Flexors.

**Starting Position:** Seated with the face placed against the two pads available, the neck flexors should be fully contracted with the head looking downward, the hands grasping the two forward hand grips, the seat should be adjusted with the face positioned against the pads so that the nose is approximately in the center of the pads.

**Description:** Lower the weight so that the neck flexors are fully stretched, pause momentarily and recover to the starting position.

**Breathing:** Inhale while lowering the weight and exhale when raising the weight.

**Points to Emphasize:**

1. All movements should be controlled, jerky movements while performing any exercise could cause injury especially while exercising the neck muscles.

2. The torso should remain erect throughout the entire exercise.

3. Proper seat alignment has not been obtained if the face is sliding on the pads available while performing the exercise.

4. 2½ pound increments should be used when 12 properly performed repetitions can be executed (a ten pound increase will probably be too much weight to perform the desired number of repetitions).

## LATERAL FLEXION

**Exercise:** Lateral Flexion.

**Equipment:** 4-Way Neck Machine.

**Starting Position:** Seated with the right side of the face resting against the two pads available, the head should be leaning to the left so that the lateral flexors on the right side of the head are fully stretched, the shoulders must remain parallel to the floor throughout the entire exercise, the torso should be erect (to isolate the left lateral flexors the athlete will mirror the above with the left side of the face resting against the pads).

**Description:** Extend the head sideward, pause momentarily and recover to the starting position.

**Breathing:** Inhale while raising the weight and exhale when lowering the weight.

**Points to Emphasize:**

    1. All movements should be controlled.

    2. When lowering the weight, a conscious effort must be made to keep the shoulders parallel with the floor.

        a. There will be an inclination to raise the shoulder in an attempt to touch the side of the head on the shoulder (if the athlete is sitting up straight and he keeps his shoulders relaxed and parallel to the floor, he will not be able to touch the head on the shoulders.

    3. The seat should be adjusted so that the flexors are taken through the full range of movement (the same seat adjustment that was used for the neck extension exercise will probably be sufficient for the lateral flexion exercise.

## WRIST CURL

**Exercise:** Wrist Curl.

**Equipment:** Multi-Exercise Machine.

**Prime Mover:** Forearm flexors.

**Starting Position:** Seated with the forearms resting on the thighs, the back of the hands are against the knees, the fingers may be extended, the knees can be elevated slightly to prevent the flexors from recovering in the contracted position.

**Description:** Flex the wrists raising the barbell forward and upward, pause momentarily and recover to the starting position.

**Breathing:** Inhale while raising the weight and exhale when recovering to the starting position.

**Points to Emphasize:**

    1. The forearm and elbow must remain in contact with the thigh to provide full range exercise.

    2. As the lifter begins to reach the point of failure, there will be a tendency to lift the forearm off the thigh when raising the weight instead of allowng the flexors to raise the weight.

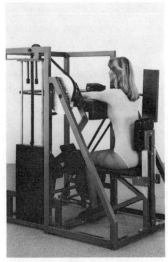

Starting position for the **Biceps Curl** on the Nautilus Biceps-Triceps Machine

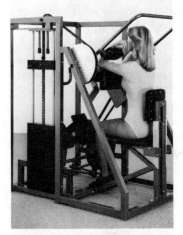

Execution of the **Biceps Curl** on the Nautilus Biceps-Triceps Machine

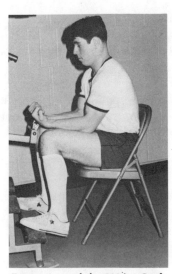

Execution of the **Wrist Curl** on the Nautilus Multi-Exercise Machine

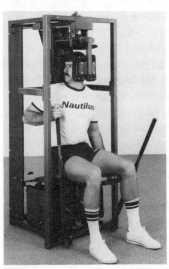

Execution of the Nautilus **Rotary Neck**

All photographs, except for the wrist curl execution, courtesy of Nautilus Sports/Medical.

## BICEPS CURL

**Exercise:** Biceps Curl.
**Equipment:** Omni Bicep Machine.
**Prime Mover:** Biceps.
**Starting Position:** Seated with the shoulders slightly below the elbows with the elbows on the pad aligned with the axis of the cam, the wrists should be placed under the wrist pads with the palms open.
**Description:** Raise the weight by flexing the arms completely while simultaneously twisting the hands (supination,) pause momentarily and recover to the starting position.
**Breathing:** Inhale while raising the weight and exhale while lowering the weight.
**Points to Emphasize:**
  1.  Do not make a fist while performing the exercise (keep the fingers extended).
  2.  Keep the head and body well back throughout the exercise.
  3.  The exercise can be performed negative only by using the legs to raise the weight and the arms to lower it.

## ROTARY NECK

**Exercise:** Rotary Neck.
**Equipment:** Rotary Neck Machine.
**Muscles Used:** Neck Rotators.
**Starting Position:** Seated with the torso erect facing away from the machine with the head secured snugly between the two pads available, the head should be rotated to the right stretching the neck muscles on the left side as much as possible.
**To Assume the Starting Position:** Sit down placing the head between the pads and adjust the pads to a snug position by pulling the overhead lever from right to left, slowly pull the right lever arm back while simultaneously twisting the head to the right until the head is fully rotated to the right.
**Breathing:** Normal.
**Points to Emphasize:**
  1.  The exercise described above is performed in a negative only fashion. However, the exercise can be performed in a normal or positive only fashion.
  2.  All movements should be controlled and performed slowly.
  3.  There should be a smooth transition from the completion of one repetition to the initiation of the next in the opposite direction.
  4.  The torso should remain erect and the shoulders stationary throughout the entire exercise.

# CHAPTER 7
## Project Total Conditioning

James A. Peterson, Ph.D.

Design of the study
Results
Thermographic diagnosis
Concurrent studies

For more than 170 years the primary mission of the United States Military Academy has been to select, train, and educate the finest of American youth to be combat arms officers in the Regular Army of the United States. An integral factor in that mission is to insure that each graduate of the Academy possesses the physical attributes necessary for leadership. To accomplish this goal every cadet is required to participate in a physical education program designed to provide him with a high level of personal fitness. To this end, one of the cornerstones of West Point's commitment to high physical standards in its graduates is a continuing, ongoing examination and evaluation of the methods used to attain such levels. Primarily because of this commitment, the Academy decided to undertake a comprehensive study of strength training and its consequences. This article provides an overview of the results of that undertaking.

The initial impetus for the direction of the study evolved from the Academy's desire to learn how to more effectively utilize the Nautilus weight training equipment it had recently purchased. With the cooperation of Col. James Anderson, Director of USMA's Office of Physical Education, representatives of Nautilus Sports/Medical Industries agreed to participate with the Academy in a joint venture. Collectively referred to as "Project Total Conditioning," the study was designed to provide USMA with the institutional knowledge of how to properly use its Nautilus equipment; to examine the relative effectiveness of different methods of strength training; and finally, (and perhaps, more importantly) to identify the consequences of a short duration, high-intensity strength training program. Answers to several questions were sought. Can significant strength gains be achieved from intense but relatively brief workouts? What effect does strength-training have on an individual's level of cardiovascular fitness?...on his degree of flexibility?...on his overall body composition? How often should an individual train to achieve maximum results? How closely should an individual be supervised to attain maximum results? What application does high-intensity strength training have to functional performance? How can the musculature of the neck be effectively strengthened? In summary, every effort was made to make "Project Total Conditioning" the most productive and inclusive field research endeavor ever undertaken in the area of strength training.


## DESIGN OF THE STUDY

Members of the Corps of Cadets served as subjects in the project. Cadets with a history of recent illness or debilitating injuries were not allowed to participate in the study. In addition, all project activities were closely monitored by physicians assigned to the US Army Hospital at West Point and by consultant physicians contracted by Nautilus. All training was prescribed and supervised by representatives of Nautilus Sports/Medical Industries. To insure project validity and objectivity, all pre- and post-training testing of the subjects was precisely controlled by Academy personnel.

In order to utilize the available personnel and resources in the most productive manner possible, several studies were concurrently conducted. The primary investigation involved the training of twenty-one (two subjects were later excused from the study because of medical reasons) varsity football players. Because this part of the project required each participant to exercise each of his body's five main muscle groups, the experimental subjects were collectively referred to as the "wholebody group". For comparative purposes, a matched control group, also consisting of intercollegiate football players, was chosen. Members of the wholebody group trained under tightly controlled conditions three times a week for a period of 8 weeks. In order to identify and help evaluate the effects of the training, an extensive battery of tests and measurements were administered to every member of both groups after the wholebody group had trained for 2 weeks and at the conclusion of the 8 week project. The pre-study testing was not scheduled until after 2 weeks of workouts had been completed in order to minimize the influence of what is commonly referred to as the "learning effect" on individual performance. In many cases of training (no matter what type of equipment is used), dramatic increases initially attained are not attributable to strength gains but rather to individual improvement in the neurological functioning of the tested muscle or muscle groups.* The pre- and post-training between-group differences provides the basis for evaluating the effects of the training.

The procedures for training were explicitly objective and precisely

---

*A review of the literature and past studies on strength training indicate that the arbitrary designation of 2 weeks of training to the "learning effect" is a generous allotment.

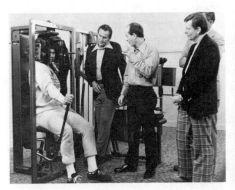

Coach Don Shula, Arthur Jones, and Dr. Robert Nirschl watch a subject train.

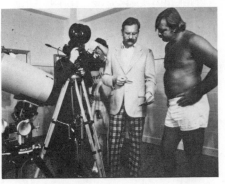

Dr. Fred Jackson explains thermographic analysis to Dick Butkus.

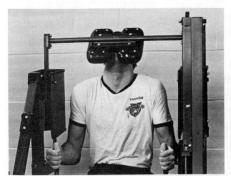

A subject exercises on the Nautilus 4-Way Neck Machine.

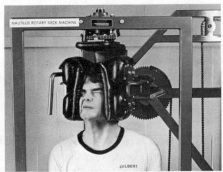

A subject exercises on the Nautilus Rotary Neck Machine.

controlled. Each subject in a wholebody group worked out at an appointed time. All training was conducted on a one-to-one basis with Nautilus personnel supervising every workout. Additional feedback regarding the program was provided by outside professionals. A number of physicians, coaches, and physical educators participated in the project as "ex-officio" consultants.* A record of each workout—the exercises performed, the amount of resistance and number of repetitions for each exercise, plus any extraneous information (e.g. illness)—was kept for every subject.

The amount of resistance and number of repetitions for the initial workouts were prescribed on the basis of an arbitrary projection of what the individual could reasonably handle. This part of the study proved to be an important factor. Even though most of the 19 wholebody group members had been working out with weights just prior to the start of the project, each subject developed severe muscular soreness after the first workout. After the first week of training, the workout program was adjusted on the basis of an individual's DEMONSTRATED performance.

Having developed the basic parameters of how to proceed with the study, the only major task remaining concerned how to accurately measure changes in strength which would result from the training. This measurement presented several problems. Even though strength is frequently identified as a basic component of physical fitness by both physicians and physical educators and is accepted by most coaches and athletes as an essential factor in athletic performance, the precise determination or expression of muscular strength is extremely difficult because of the variety of conditions which can effect such a determination. Perhaps the two most dominant of these conditions are: 1) the mechanical advantage produced by the body's system of levers, and 2) the influence of neurological factors. First of all, since all contractions express their forces through the movements of skeletal levers, the end product is a measurement of movement of force (or torque) rather than force per se. As a result, the position of the levers involved in a specific exercise becomes important. The angle of attachment effects both the strength of a muscle and its resultant mechanical advantage. To offer a basic example of this, all other factors being equal, an individual with relatively short arms can biceps-curl more resistance than a man with longer arms because of his mechanical (angular) advantage.

A second complicating factor in strength measurements evolves from the fact muscles respond to stimulation from the nervous system. As a

*One of the primary purposes for the participation by Nautilus personnel in "Project Total Conditioning" was to evaluate several prototype machines which were used in the study. These "consultants" aided this cause.

result, maximum volitional strength is greatly affected by neurological factors.* Unfortunately, no one has been able to precisely identify or quantify the influence of these factors. The literature, however, suggests several viable alternatives. If a reasonable amount of training is alloted for initial learning effect (as was done in "Project Total Conditioning"), absolute strength can be measured by the use of a device known as a tensiometer. On the other hand if tensiometers are unavailable, relative strength changes can be inferred from the ability of an individual to lift an increased amount of resistance the approximate same number of times for any given exercise. Other plausible methods for inferring strength increase concern quantifying the amount of lean muscle mass in an individual and measuring an individual's ability to perform on a functional item which involves strength (e.g. leg power). In an attempt to provide a maximum amount of information on the consequences of the Nautilus strength training, "Project Total Conditioning" incorporated each of the four alternatives as a means to identify strength changes.

A series of tensiometers (involving the major muscle groups of the body) was developed. Tensiometers are instruments which measure the force an individual can exert at a specific point in the range of motion. By means of an attached dynamometer, the force (pressure) an individual exerts against a static resistance is quantified. Six machines—each designed to be compatible with the movement required in a Nautilus machine of a comparable function—were used: 1)Bench Press; 2) Leg Extension; 3) Leg Curl; 4) Hip and Back; 5) Biceps Curl; and 6) One for each of the four basic functions of the neck. While the mechanical advantage offered by a tensiometer set at a fixed position might vary slightly from individual to individual, it would not change for the individual himself. In other words, although one subject might have a slightly more disadvantageous angle of rotation than another on a specific tensiometer, the resultant pre- and post-measurements reflect valid change since the angle remains constant from test to test for each individual. Unfortunately, although steps were taken to insure repeatability on the tensiometer measuring, numerous operational problems were encountered regarding the use of these machines. Except for the information furnished by the neck tensiometer, the data provided by the tensiometers was inaccurate and was subsequently discarded.

---

*The term "neurological factors" also includes "psychological factors," such as motivation. Collectively, members of the Corps of Cadets are a motivated and disciplined group. The objectivity of the assessment that the subjects were motivated was also strongly supported by the outside individuals who were contracted to do the ergometer testing. Refer to the CARDIOVASCULAR FITNESS section in this article for additional information.

Another study examined the consequences of multi-functional, bilateral neck-strength training. Sixteen varsity football players engaged in a neck strengthening program using only the three Nautilus neck machines. The results of these subjects were compared with those achieved by a control group whose members participated in a semi-supervised neck strengthening program of isometric exercises devised by the USMA football staff.

Two secondary studies involved members of the Academy's club squad rugby and volleyball teams. Rugby team members were solicited as subjects in a study designed to examine the effects on overall neck strength of a twice weekly versus a three-times weekly workout program. In the second project, twenty-two volleyball team members volunteered to participate in an investigation designed to compare the effects on vertical jumping ability of a strengthening program which utilizes the Nautilus regular hip and back machine versus one which uses the Nautilus DUOsymmetric POLY-contractile hip and back machine.

In order to systematically present and discuss the results of "Project Total Conditioning" in as logical and comprehensively a manner as possible, the findings have been categorized into seven (separate but interrelated) subsections: 1) strength training; 2) neck strengthening; 3) cardiovascular fitness; 4) flexibility; 5) body composition; 6) thermographic diagnosis; and 7) concurrent studies.

## RESULTS

### STRENGTH TRAINING

In the past twenty years, coaches, athletes, and physical educators have been increasingly aware of the role of strength in sport and athletic performance. Unfortunately, there are still many unknown factors regarding the acquisition and maintenance of strength. (Strength may generally be defined as the muscular force exerted against movable and immovable objects). An overview of the considerable volume of literature devoted to the topic reveals a wide disparity in identifying the proper way to train and the consequences of such training. "Project Total Conditioning" was designed to provide a solution to some of the enigmas associated with strength training.

Two of the most widely debated aspects of strength-training concern the intensity of training which is necessary to achieve maximum results and the length of time which should be devoted to training. In the present study, nineteen subjects trained three days a week on alternate days, with a two day rest after the third workout, for a period of 8 weeks. Contrary to traditional practices (and/or misconceptions) each workout

Table 7-1. Exercises and machines used in "PROJECT TOTAL CONDITIONING"

| EXERCISE | MACHINE |
|---|---|
| 1. Leg Extension | Compound Leg |
| 2. Leg Press | Compound Leg |
| 3. Squat | Leg and Back |
| 4. Hip and Back | Super Hip and Back DUO-POLY Hip and Back |
| 5. Leg Curl | Leg Curl |
| 6. Pullover | Pullover |
| 7. Bench Press | Infimetric Bench Omni Bench |
| 8. Chins | Multi-Exercise |
| 9. Dips | Multi-Exercise |
| 10. Torso Arm Pulldown | Torso Arm |

| EXERCISE | MACHINE |
|---|---|
| 11. Seated Press | DUO - Shoulder |
| 12. Double Chest | Double Chest |
| 13. Decline Press | Double Chest |
| 14. Biceps Curl | Curl-Triceps DUO-POLY Curl |
| 15. Triceps Curl | Curl-Triceps DUO-POLY Triceps |
| 16. Neck Extension | 4 - Way Neck |
| 17. Neck Flexion | 4 - Way Neck |
| 18. Bi-lateral Neck Flexion | 4 - Way Neck |
| 19. Shoulder Shrug | Neck and Shoulder |
| 20. Rotary Neck | Rotary Neck |

was relatively brief in duration. Each subject was required to move from exercise to exercise with a minimum of recovery time between exercises. For all practical purposes, the intensity of the workouts was so severe that it would have been impossible to appreciably extend them. During the first workouts a few of the subjects became nauseated, but after several weeks of training, not only had such negative reactions entirely disappeared, but the average time to complete a comparable workout had been considerably shortened.

The normal workout consisted of ten basic exercises. In addition, twice a week, the wholebody group workouts included six exercises designed to strengthen the neck. Table 1 lists the exercises (along with the required equipment) which, in varying combinations, constituted the training program. Table 2 lists the "typical" workout program which was followed.

Three different ways of exercising were prescribed. In the first method, an exercise was done in NORMAL fashion (the subject lifts and lowers the weight under his own power). In the second type of training, an exercise was performed in a NEGATIVE-ACCENTUATED fashion (e.g. the subject lifts the weight with two limbs and lowers the weight using only one limb). In effect, negative-accentuated work, as opposed to "normal work", doubles the amount of weight which can be lowered with one extremity (arm or leg). The final (and perhaps most strenuous) way of exercising was doing exercises in a NEGATIVE-ONLY fashion. In this method experimenter personnel lifted the resistance to the contracted (concentric contraction) position for the subject who in turn was required to lower the weight at a controlled pace through the eccentric contraction phase of a muscle's range of motion. The primary advantage of negative-only exercising is that it greatly increases the amount of resistance that an individual can handle since quite obviously an individual can lower considerably more weight than he can raise. In a program designed to exercise only in a "normal fashion," the resistance in the eccentric phase is by definition limited to the amount of weight lifted by the amount of weight lifted in the concentric part of muscle contraction.

Although reliable tensiometer measurements were not obtained in some cases, it is still possible to observe the strength increases which were produced by the training. Tables 3 and 4 illustrate the significant nature of these changes. By comparing the average amount of resistance that an individual used for identical* workouts—one at the beginning of

---

*Identical with respect to the exercises performed, the order of the exercises, and the relative intensity of the workout.

Table 7-2. The workout program for the wholebody group for "PROJECT TOTAL CONDITIONING"

| Exercise[1] | DAY 1 | 2 | 3 | 4 | 5 | 6 | 7 | 8 | 9 | 10 | 11 | 12 | 13 | 14 | 15 | 16 | 17 |
|---|---|---|---|---|---|---|---|---|---|---|---|---|---|---|---|---|---|
| 1. Leg Extension | | R | | R | R | | R | R | R | R | R | NA | R | NA | R | R | |
| 2. Leg Press | | R | | R | R | | R | R | R | R | R | NA | R | NA | R | R | R |
| 3. Squat | R | | R | | R | R | | R | | R | | | R | | | | R |
| 4. Super Hip & Back | NA | NA | NA | | R | NA | | | | | | NA | | NO | | | NA |
| 5. Duo-Poly Hip & Back | | R | | R | | | R | R | R | R | R | | R | | R | R | |
| 6. Leg Curl | NA | NA | NA | NA | R | NA | NA | R | NA | R | R | NA | R | NA | R | NA | NA |
| 7. Pullover | NA | NA | NA | NA | R | NA | | R | | | R | NA | R | NO | R | NA | NA |
| 8. Duo-Poly Pullover | | R | | R | | R | R | | R | R | | | R | | | R | |
| 9. Chins[2] | R/NO | | R/NO | | R/NO | NO | | R/NO | NO | NO | R/NO | NO | R/NO | NO | NO | | NO |
| 10. Omni Bench | NO | NA | NO | NA | R | NO | NA | R | NO | NA | R | NO | R | NO | R | NA | NO |
| 11. Dips[2] | R/NO | | R/NO | | R/NO | NO | | R/NO | NO | NO | R/NO | NO | R/NO | NO | NO | | NO |
| 12. BNTA[3] | R | R | R | R | R | R | R | R | | R | R | | R | | | R | R |
| 13. Seated Press | | R | | R | R | | R | R | | | | | R | | R | R | |
| 14. Double Chest | R | | R | | R | R | | R | | | | R | R | R | R | R | |
| 15. Duo-Poly Curl | | R | | R | R | | R | R | | | | | R | | | | |
| 16. Duo-Poly Tricep | R | R | | R | R | | R | R | | | | | R | | | | |
| 17. Curl-Tricep | | | | | | | | | R | | R | R | R | R | R | R | |
| 18. 4-Way Neck | R | | | R | R | | | | R | | R | R | R | R | R | R | R |
| 19. Shrug | R | | R | R | R | R | | R | R | | R | R | R | R | | R | R |
| 20. Rotary Neck | R | | R | R | R | R | | R | R | | R | R | R | R | | R | R |

KEY: R = Regular (normal) fashion; NO = Negative only fashion; NA = Negative-accentuated fashion

[1] The order of exercises which was generally followed corresponded to the descending numerical order #1-20.

[2] For both the chins and the dips, there were several workouts where the subject was required to perform 10 repetitions. In most instances, the subject could not execute 10 proper reps in normal fashion. In those cases, he completed his set of 10 by doing negative-only reps.

[3] BNTA = Behind the Neck Torso Arm

the training, the other at the conclusion of the 8 week period—the difference can logically be attributed to a change in strength. Such a conclusion can be given additional credence when the 2 weeks of training which were allocated to "learning" are considered.

Over a period of 6 weeks, the 18 wholebody subjects increased the amount of resistance used in their first two workouts* of the training by an average of 58.54% and 43.06% respectively. The variance in the amount of change incurred by the two "sets" of workouts (15.48%) can primarily be attributed to differences in the programs used for the first and second days of training. The program for the 1st and 17th workouts included one set of each of the following exercises: squat, hip and back, leg curl, pullover, chins, dips, omni bench, torso arm, double chest, and decline press. In the 2nd and 16th workouts, a set of the leg extension, leg press, seated press, duo-poly curl, and duo-poly triceps was substituted for the squat, chins, dips, double chest, and decline press exercises.

Despite the dramatic changes achieved by even the lowest man (improvement-wise), there were circumstances attendant to the project which undoubtedly prevented even greater levels of improvement. During the first 4 weeks of training for record, each subject participated in spring football practice. Quite possibly, the energy expenditure for spring practice not only minimized some of the gains produced by the strength training but also precluded additional increases by limiting the amount of rest (and resultant recovery ability) available to each man. Further demands on the time and energies of each subject were incurred by the final academic exam schedule which was held concurrent with the last week of training. In addition, a few subjects missed several workouts (or trained at less than full effort) because of minor injuries or illnesses. One subject contracted the mumps but remained in the project anyway. His missing three full workouts undoubtedly accounts for his comparatively poor showing among the wholebody group members (he ranked last on the 1st/17th comparison and 10th on the other).

An examination of Tables 3 and 4 reveals another meaningful statistic: the subjects, not only significantly increased their level of strength, but DECREASED the time required to go through an identical workout. Despite a slight increase in the number of average repetitions performed each workout, the duration of the training dropped over 9 minutes and

---

*Comparisons were only made of the 1st and 17th, 2nd and 16th workouts because of spatial reasons and because they were among the few times that an exact workout was repeated.

Table 7-3. A comparison of the 1st and 17th workouts of the wholebody group subjects.

| Subject (a) | 1st WORKOUT | | | 17th WORKOUT (c) | | | NET CHANGE | |
|---|---|---|---|---|---|---|---|---|
| | Ave Wt. (10 exercises) | Ave No. of Reps | Duration (b) (in Min) | Ave Wt. (10 exercises) | Ave No. of Reps | Duration (in Min) | Ave Wt. (in Lbs) | Change (%) |
| 1. | 99.0 | 9.3 | N.A. | 168.0 | 10.4 | N.A. | 69.0 | 69.70 |
| 2. | 80.5 | 6.7 | 49 | 135.5 | 9.2 | 25 | 55.0 | 68.32 |
| 3. | 96.5 | 7.8 | 42 | 160.5 | 8.3 | 27 | 64.0 | 66.32 |
| 4. | 93.0 | 8.0 | 43 | 154.0 | 8.9 | 22 | 61.0 | 65.59 |
| 5. | 80.5 | 9.3 | N.A. | 132.0 | 9.2 | N.A. | 51.5 | 63.98 |
| 6. | 91.5 | 7.3 | 29 | 149.0 | 8.7 | 21 | 57.5 | 62.77 |
| 7. | 98.5 | 11.0 | 33 | 157.5 | 8.8 | 30 | 59.0 | 59.90 |
| 8. | 101.0 | 9.7 | 44.5 | 161.5 | 10.7 | 35 | 60.5 | 59.90 |
| 9. | 98.0 | 10.5 | 33 | 156.5 | 10.8 | 30 | 58.5 | 59.69 |
| 10. (d) | 95.0 | 9.7 | 33 | 150.5 | 8.7 | 38 | 55.5 | 58.42 |
| 11. | 94.0 | 7.9 | N.A. | 147.5 | 10.0 | N.A. | 53.5 | 56.91 |
| 12. | 101.5 | 7.3 | N.A. | 159.0 | 8.2 | N.A. | 57.5 | 56.65 |
| 13. | 88.5 | 9.2 | 35 | 137.5 | 9.0 | 29 | 49.0 | 55.37 |
| 14. (d) | 89.5 | 13.7 | 34 | 138.5 | 11.4 | 30 | 49.0 | 54.75 |
| 15. | 94.0 | 8.2 | N.A. | 142.0 | 9.0 | N.A. | 48.0 | 51.06 |
| 16. | 104.5 | 8.6 | N.A. | 157.0 | 10.4 | N.A. | 52.5 | 50.24 |
| 17. | 97.0 | 9.8 | 40 | 144.0 | 10.8 | 28 | 52.5 | 50.24 |
| 18. | 85.5 | 9.1 | N.A. | 124.5 | 11.5 | N.A. | 39.0 | 45.61 |
| Mean = | 93.78 | 9.06 | 37.73 | 148.61 | 9.67 | 28.64 | 54.83 | 58.54 |

a. Arranged in rank order by achieved percentage of improvement. Only 18 subjects are listed even though 19 participated in the study because one subject was injured during football practice and was subsequently excused from some exercises.

b. Rounded off to the nearest half minute. N.A. is used to designate those for whom no recording of the duration of their workout is available.

c. The 17th workout was the last workout. The 18th workout was ommitted because of scheduling problems.

d. Subject's #10 and #14 pre-scores are based on workout #3. Both were recovering from injuries suffered at spring football practice and did not engage in the program used for the 17th workout until the 3rd workout.

Table 7-4. A comparison of the 2nd and 16th workouts of the wholebody group subjects. (a)

| Subject (a) | 2nd WORKOUT Ave Wt. (10 exercises) | Ave No. of Reps | Duration (in Min) | 16th WORKOUT Ave Wt. (10 exercises) | Ave No. of Reps | Duration (in Min) | NET CHANGE Ave Wt. (in Lbs) | Change (%) |
|---|---|---|---|---|---|---|---|---|
| 1. | 60.3 | 9.4 | 26 | 96.0 | 14.6 | 25 | 35.7 | 59.20 |
| 2. | 75.5 | 14.4 | 31 | 114.0 | 12.1 | 23.5 | 38.5 | 50.99 |
| 3. | 74.5 | 13.0 | 36 | 112.3 | 13.7 | 34 | 37.8 | 50.74 |
| 4. | 68.5 | 11.9 | 31 | 103.0 | 12.3 | 21.5 | 34.5 | 50.36 |
| 5. | 78.5 | 13.3 | 23 | 115.8 | 13.6 | 23 | 37.3 | 47.52 |
| 6. | 72.0 | 11.9 | 30 | 105.5 | 12.4 | 24 | 33.5 | 46.53 |
| 7. | 75.0 | 10.7 | 37 | 109.3 | 13.7 | 31 | 34.3 | 45.73 |
| 8. | 72.5 | 13.3 | 35 | 103.0 | 12.2 | 23 | 30.5 | 42.07 |
| 9. | 61.5 | 9.4 | 21 | 87.3 | 13.3 | 26 | 25.8 | 41.95 |
| 10. (b) | 66.5 | 13.3 | 26 | 94.0 | 13.2 | 22.5 | 27.5 | 41.35 |
| 11. | 77.5 | 21.5 | 44 | 109.0 | 12.2 | 22 | 31.5 | 40.65 |
| 12. | 71.3 | 12.9 | 25 | 100.0 | 10.5 | 20 | 28.7 | 40.25 |
| 13. | 80.3 | 11.8 | N.A. | 112.0 | 13.1 | N.A. | 31.7 | 39.48 |
| 14. | 71.3 | 10.7 | 24 | 99.0 | 11.5 | 18 | 27.7 | 38.85 |
| 15. | 76.5 | 16.9 | 33 | 106.0 | 15.5 | 28 | 29.5 | 38.56 |
| 16. | 72.5 | 10.6 | 34 | 97.5 | 10.7 | 38 | 25.0 | 34.48 |
| 17. | 82.3 | 10.9 | 23 | 11.03 | 10.6 | 19 | 28.0 | 34.02 |
| 18. | 72.5 | 9.1 | 23.5 | 96.0 | 11.7 | 19 | 23.5 | 32.41 |
| Mean = | 72.7 | 12.5 | 27.92 | 103.9 | 12.6 | 23.19 | 31.2 | 43.06 |

a. The program used for the 2nd and 16th workouts differed from the one prescribed for the 1st and 17th days of training.

b. Subject #11's data for the 2nd workout is based on his 4th workout. He did not participate in the program used for the 16th workout until #4 because of training.

144

4.5 minutes respectively from the expended times for the initial two periods. The nine minute decrease might have been even larger.

By the 17th workout, all of the subjects had to put on a device which would accommodate additional weight for both the chins and the dips. In the initial workout this strap was not needed. When the fact that the entire 6 week program involved less than 8.5 hours of actual training per man is considered, the significant increases in strength and decreases in the duration of the workouts appear to be even more noteworthy.

In order to provide a measure of the functional application of the training, three items were administered to each member of both the wholebody and the control groups: 2-mile run (wind, stamina), 40-yard dash (speed), and vertical jump (leg power). These items were chosen because of their somewhat universal acceptance (by football coaches) as integral components of the skills required to play football. Table 5 illustrates that on each of the three measures, the wholebody group subjects improved their performance MORE than did the control group members.

The differences between the two groups on the functional items were substantial. The wholebody subject's level of improvement was more than four times that achieved by members of the control group on both the 2-mile run (4.32 x) and the vertical jump (4.57 x). On the 40-yard dash the wholebody group improved 1.89 times the rate of the control group. The significant increase produced in vertical jumping ability is consistent with the gains achieved in leg strength by the wholebody subjects. The dramatic changes which occurred over a period of only 6 weeks in the 2-mile run times will be examined in greater detail in the section on cardiovascular fitness. One final point to consider in this section concerns the relatively moderate degree of improvement in the times for the 40-yard dash. This occurrence can be at least partially attributed to the fact that prior to the advent of training, members of both groups used the 40-yard dash as an integral part of their conditioning program to prepare for spring football practice. Once "Project Total Conditioning" and spring practice began, this specificity training (doing 40-yard dashes) by-and-large ended.

## NECK STRENGTHENING

In light of the overwhelming number of neck injuries which result from athletic competition, it is essential that both coaches and athletes undertake steps to strengthen the musculature of the neck (and surrounding shoulder area). All individuals who participate in sports which involve forceful displacement and contact of either the head or the neck should include neck strengthening exercises as an integral part

## Table 7-5. A comparison of wholebody group vs control group performance on 3 functional measures.

TWO MILE RUN (a)

|  | Pre-Training (in min) | Post-Training (in min) | Mean Difference (in sec) | Improvement (%) |
|---|---|---|---|---|
| Wholebody Group ( N = 19 ) | 13:18 | 11:50 | 88 | 11.02 |
| Control Group ( N = 15 ) | 13:04 | 12:44 | 20 | 2.55 |

FORTY YARD DASH (b)

|  | Pre-Training (in seconds) | Post-Training (in seconds) | Mean Difference (in seconds) | Improvement (%) |
|---|---|---|---|---|
| Wholebody Group ( N = 19 ) | 5.1467 | 5.0933 | 0.0534 | 1.04 |
| Control Group ( N = 15 ) | 4.7933 | 4.7667 | 0.0266 | 0.55 |

VERTICAL JUMP (c)

|  | Pre-Training ( in inches) | Post-Training (in inches) | Mean Difference (in inches) | Improvement (%) |
|---|---|---|---|---|
| Wholebody Group ( N = 19 ) | 22.600 | 24.067 | 1.467 | 6.49 |
| Control Group ( N = 15 ) | 21.692 | 22.000 | 0.308 | 1.42 |

a. Run on a tartan, indoor track.

b. Best of one trial, run in tennis shoes, administered in the gymnasium.

c. Best of three trials, one hand reach.

of their conditioning program. Unfortunately, in many strength training programs, this aspect of self-improvement has been accorded (at best) minimal attention. In fact, the two most apparent overriding common-alities which can be identified as existing between the "traditional" methods of strengthening the neck—calisthenic-type exercises such as bridging, the buddy-system of exercising (one individual pushes against a resistance provided by someone else); and the use of external para-phernalia, such as harness straps which accommodate free weights, etc. —are: 1) such methods generally are very awkward and as a result, inhibit proper form; and 2) these "programs" typically produce less than desired-for results.

In "Project Total Conditioning," efforts were made to minimize the first aforementioned limitation, thereby abrogating the second concern. Three machines—each designed to enable an individual to exercise the neck in proper form for the basic functions of the neck—were used. For comparative pusposes, the subjects who participated in this part of the study were placed into three groups.* The first group consisted of the 19 wholebody subjects discussed in the previous section. In two of their three weekly workouts, these individuals included exercises for streng-thening their necks. The second group was designated as the "neck-only" group because the sixteen individuals in this bracket restricted their strength training to the muscles of the neck and shoulders. The last group was comprised of 14 members who served as a "control" group. Subjects in the control group did not participate in the training conducted during the project. Any exercising these individuals did was done either on their own or under the auspices of the USMA football staff.

The program for strengthening the neck consisted of three weekly workouts for the neck-only group and two neck sessions for the whole-body subjects. One basic program was used for all neck-training workouts. This program required each subject to perform one set of six exercises: shoulder shrug, neck rotation (rotary neck), and the exercises done on the 4-way neck machine (flexion, extension, lateral flexion-right, and lateral flexion-left). When an individual was able to do 12 repetitions of an exercise, except for the rotary neck which remained constant at 12 repetitions (six each direction), the amount of resistance was increased to the next higher increment. Each participant took approximately 8 minutes to complete a "neck" workout during the initial stages and less than seven minutes thereafter.

*All of the subjects who were part of this section were members of the intercollegiate football team.

Similar to the procedures discussed in the section on the wholebody strength training, the first 2 weeks of exercising were devoted to the "learning effect." Training-for-record started at the sixth workout. Table 6 represents the between group differences which resulted from 6 weeks of training.

The subjects in both the wholebody and the neck-only groups increased their relative neck strength (91.92% and 56.72% respectively) at a greater level than did the control group members (27.84%). These significant changes are even more substantial when the fact that they were achieved in approximately two hours of actual training is considered. The large variance between the results achieved by the wholebody and the neck-only groups is at least partially attributable to the amount of supervision members of each group received during training. The wholebody group was closely supervised AT ALL TIMES, insuring that each subject performed EVERY repetition in proper form. As a concession to experimenter manpower requirements and in an attempt to ascertain (to at least a peripheral degree) the influence of experimenter supervision, the neck-only subjects received only minimal input from an instructor during their actual training. Their progress and form were monitored and charted, but only on infrequent occasions were the neck-only subjects "pushed" to the apparent limit of their capabilities by an experimenter. The improvement attained by the control group members is the result of a combination of the effects of engaging in spring football practice with its attendant "involvement" of the neck and lifting on their own initiative.

The neck circumference results are somewhat more difficult to evaluate. By any rational criterion, the subjects who participated in the Nautilus training increased the size of their necks by a significant degree. However, the direction of the variance between the wholebody and the neck-only groups is inconsistent with both the tensiometer measurements and the personal observations of those personnel involved with "Project Total Conditioning." By all reasonable expectations, the neck of each of the wholebody subjects should have increased in size substantially more than those of the neck-only group. The recorded differences are apparently the result of operational complications. The same individuals did not measure the necks of the wholebody subjects who calculated the neck-only and control group figures. In addition, a slightly different measuring instrument was used to obtain the wholebody data. Complicating the dilemma was the fact that the wholebody circumference measurements were not available for analysis until after the project had been completed. While the neck-only and control group measurements were conducted by Academy personnel, the responsibility of securing the wholebody group calculations was

Table 7-6. A comparison of the results of the neck strengthening program. (a)

**TENSIOMETER STRENGTH (b)**

| | Pre-Training | Post-Training | Mean Difference | Improvement (%) |
|---|---|---|---|---|
| Wholebody Group (N = 18) | 586.28 | 1,125.16 | 538.88 | 91.92 |
| Neck-Only Group (N = 16) | 571.06 | 894.94 | 323.88 | 56.72 |
| Control Group (N = 16) | 620.50 | 793.25 | 172.75 | 27.84 |

**NECK CIRCUMFERENCE (c)**

| | Pre-Training (in inches) | Post-Training (in inches) | Mean Difference (in inches) | Improvement (%) |
|---|---|---|---|---|
| Wholebody Group (N = 49) | 16.38 | 16.82 | + 0.44 | 2.67 |
| Neck-Only Group (N = 16) | 16.28 | 17.03 | + 0.75 | 4.61 |
| Control Group (N = 14) | 16.47 | 16.62 | + 0.15 | 0.91 |

a. The pre- post-test data on the average amount lifted and number of repetitions performed is not presented because the neck-only group subject trained in a semi-supervised environment. As such, their recorded number of properly performed repetitions could, in some instances, be inaccurate.

b. The totals reflect the sum of four tensiometer measurements — one each for extension, flexion, lateral flexion — left, and lateral flexion — right. The scores on one of the wholebody subjects was ommitted because he was sick on the day the testing was conducted.

c. No pre-training measurement was taken for two control group subjects.

149

assigned to outside personnel who were involved with another aspect of the project.

A few wholebody subjects were measured DURING the course of the 6 weeks of training by the same individuals who conducted the testing of the other groups. In EVERY single case, the resultant measurements of the wholebody subjects indicated that the AVERAGE increase in neck circumference for the nineteen wholebody group members would exceed at least one inch by the end of the training.* Although the existing discrepancies in the circumference data cannot be resolved, the unabated fact remains that significant increases in neck strength were produced by both the wholebody and the neck-only group training.

## CARDIOVASCULAR FITNESS

Cardiovascular fitness is an integral component of both an individual's level of overall physical fitness and an individual's capability for sustained athletic performance. A brief review of the basic function of the circulatory system can clarify these basic assumptions. The primary function of the circulatory system may be stated in one simple word— "transport." It transports essentials like oxygen and glucose to the cells, and by-products, such as carbon dioxide, from the cells. As would be expected, the circulatory system is called upon to increase its transport of essentials to the cells and of waste products from the cells during muscular exertion. This need, of course, is directly related to the intensity and duration of exertion. It follows that one of the limiting factors in athletics and sport is the ability of this system to meet the demands imposed by the body during competition. Therefore two of the benefits which can be derived from a functionally efficient circulatory system are an improved capacity for work (exercise) and an increased ability to perform the transport function.

Traditionally, physicians and exercise physiologists have held that participation in strength training does not increase an individual's capacity to meet the "transport" (oxygen-in—$CO_2$-out) requirements of strenuous exercise. Although this capacity is collectively known by various names, this section refers to it by one of its most common desig-

---

*Similar operational problems occurred during the measurement of skin-fold thickness and body fat percentages. In the case of skin-fold data, however, calculations on each member of ALL three groups were obtained by the same experimenter.

nations—"cardiovascular (C.V.) fitness."* Numerous researchers have found that the individual who wishes to improve his C.V. capacity by means of an exercise program must incorporate several factors into his efforts. The program must be of sufficient intensity to have the heart rate of the participant reach a level of at least 145-150 beats per minute;** this rate should be sustained for a minimum of 10-12 minutes; and the participant should engage in such exercising 3-4 times a week (the literature is equivocal on the exact number of times).

Conventional strength training practices have prevented C.V. improvement from occurring because even on those occasions when a sufficiently higher heart rate is attained by a participant, such a rate is typically not sustained for more than a brief period. In the present study, an attempt was made to train the wholebody subjects in such a manner that improvement in their overall level of cardiovascular fitness would occur. By limiting the rest period between the exercises to a few seconds and by preventing the subjects from resting during the actual training, a high degree of intensity was achieved and maintained for the duration of the workout.

In order to ascertain the effects of the training, several tests were administered—on a pre- post-training basis—to both the wholebody and the control group members. Differences on the initial test date were determined by a T-test for each variable. If there were no initial significant differences, then the T-test was applied to the post-training data to determine the effects of the training. If there were significant differences on the initial data, then analysis of covariance was used to determine the relative degree of any changes which occurred between the two groups as a result of the training.

Three different states of the cardiovascular function were examined: 1) C.V. capacity at rest; 2) responses to sub-maximal work; and 3) responses to maximal work. The tests for the resting state consisted of measuring each subjects heart rate (HR), systolic (blood is being forced out of the heart) blood pressure (SBP), diastolic (the chambers of the heart are filling with blood) blood pressure (DBP), and systolic tension time index—an accepted measure of coronary circulation which is calculated by multiplying heart rate x systolic blood pressure (STTI).

An evaluation of the effects on the sub-maximal state was achieved by having each subject perform on a Bodyguard model 990 bicycle

---

*Cardio refers to the "heart" and the vascular portion consists of the large arteries, the small arteries, the arterioles leading to the tissues, and the capillaries within the tissues.

**In general, the more of the body's large musculature involved in the exercise, the easier it will be to reach a heart rate of 145-150 beats per minute.

ergometer. An ergometer is a basic research instrument which allows a subject to pedal against a resistance (load) which can be predetermined and adjusted (when necessary) by the experimenter. The sub-maximal tests required each subject to perform a continuous, progressive ergometer ride with increasing work loads (360 kpm/min increase) every two minutes until the subject could no longer sustain the rate (60 rpm) or wanted to stop. This was followed by two minutes at the initial light load (360 kpm/min), then three minutes of rest. At each condition, the HR, SBP, DBP, STTI, and a subjective rating (by the subject) of his perceived exertion (RPE) were obtained. Cardiac feedback was provided by means of a continuous EKG which was obtained on each subject while on the ergometer. The maximal state was evaluated by means of two measures: total riding time and 2-mile run performance.*

The results of the testing were conclusive. On NONE of the 60 indices purporting to evaluate the effects of the training on the cardiovascular function was the control group better on the final testing period (or on the change from initial to final) than the wholebody group. The following significant differences (.05 level**) were caused by the training afforded to the wholebody group: Lower HR at 360, 1080, 1260, 1620, and 1800 kpm/min; lower STTI at 360, and RPE at 1260; a higher amount of work necessary before the subject achieved a heart rate of 170; a longer ride time; and a lower time required to run 2 miles. These calculations mean that the training caused the players to work more efficiently (lower HR) at light, moderate and near maximal levels. They could also do more work before reaching a heart rate of 170, as well as more total work. Their improvement in their 2-mile run performances also indicates that they were less stressed at maximal levels. For the coach and the athlete, the implication is clear: these subjects could perform at a more efficient rate for a longer period of time. In the athletic arena, where contests are frequently decided by inches or other fractions, such training could play an important role.

---

*With the exception of administering the 2-mile run test, all cardiovascular testing was conducted by outside consultants. In light of the fact that these individuals were not informed until after all testing had been completed about which subjects were a member of which group—control or wholebody, their efforts can be accorded an additional degree of legitimacy.

**Many researchers frequently use .05 as the level of significance. It means that the differences can be accepted with 95% degree of certainty as having occurred as a result of the special training.

## FLEXIBILITY

In any examination of the factors that effect human physical performance, consideration must be given to flexibility. Basically, flexibility can be defined as the degree to which a joint is free to move throughout its normal range of motion. The primary determinant in flexibility is the musculature surrounding a specific joint. If the muscles and tendons encircling a joint are required on a regular basis to stretch—to elongate—through a normal range of motion, the joint will maintain a normal level of flexibility. On the other hand, when the muscles surrounding a joint are not regularly required to make normal range adjustments, a shortening of that musculature will develop, and a loss of flexibility will occur.

The fear that "tightened" muscles result in a lack of flexibility undoubtedly accounts for much of the superstition and misconception regarding the relationships between strength training and flexibility. Many coaches and athletes have not adopted strength training into their conditioning programs because an erroneous belief that all such training will result in the participant becoming "muscle-bound." The assumption is made by these individuals that if a person has bulging muscles, he must have sacrificed some degree of flexibility. The truth of the matter is that, with proper training methods, normal flexibility will not only be uneffected, but may even be increased by strength training.

When planning a program the principles which should be considered are: 1) for each exercise, a muscle should be stretched through a full range of motion; and 2) both the agonist and the antagonist should receive comparable attention in any strength program. Muscles are set up in opposing pairs around joints. In a discussion of elbow flexion, for example, the biceps is the agonist, or the muscle responsible for the action being considered. The triceps, which in this case would be the muscle "opposing" this action, is called the antagonist. These designations are solely based on the specific joint movement being considered. If, however, attention was focused on elbow extension rather than on flexion, the triceps would be referred to as the agonist and the biceps as the antagonist. In order to avoid a loss in flexibility, strength training programs should be balanced to give equitable attention to the development of both the antagonists and the agonists of a particular muscle group.

In "Project Total Conditioning," steps were undertaken to comply with both principles. By design, the machines required each subject to both fully stretch and perform each exercise through the normal range of motion. In addition, the workouts were planned to give an appropriate amount of attention to each of the agonist-antagonist pairs of the major muscle groups.

The procedures for examining the effects of the training on flexibility were similar to those discussed in earlier sections of this article. Because of their potential import for human (and in particular, athletic) performance, four measures of flexibility—trunk extension, trunk flexion, and shoulder flexion—were selected for examination. Subjects in both the wholebody and the control groups were tested on a pre- and post-training basis on each of the four items. The relative degree of changes on the four items over the 6 week period of the study provides the basis for identifying the effects of the training.

Table 7 illustrates the fact that the training produced significant changes in flexibility. On each of the tested measures, the wholebody group achieved a substantially higher degree of improvement than did the control group.*

The results provide formidable support for the contention that strength training, when properly performed, can in fact increase flexibility. In a period of only 6 weeks, the wholebody group subjects improved on the three flexibility measures by an average of almost 11% (10.92). In contrast, the average gain in flexibility for the control group members was less than 1% (0.85).

## BODY COMPOSITION

Body fat is accepted by researchers as the major storage form of energy. On the other hand, there have been a number of studies which indicate that excessive body fat can have a debilitating effect on human performance, individual health, and psychological well-being. For the athlete, unwanted body fat serves as an unneeded obstacle which can hinder his competitive efforts.

There is an abundance of evidence to support the conclusion that in order to reduce fat, it is necessary to expend more calories than are consumed. Traditionally, strength training has not been considered to be an activity which would greatly facilitate such a "negative calorie balance." In "Project Total Conditioning," steps were undertaken to identify the effects of high-intensity, brief duration training on body fat measurements. Two types of body fat calculations were obtained. A relative percentage of body fat for each subject as determined by a machine known as the Whole Body Counter and skin-fold measurements.

Prior to the first workout of training-for-record and at the conclusion

---

* Only the results from three flexibility measures are presented in Table 7. The data on the shoulder flexion was obtained through the coordinated use of synchronized photography and a goniometer (an instrument to measure the degree of angle) and was not available at the press time for this article.

## Table 7-7. A comparison of the effects of training on flexibility.

**TRUNK EXTENSION**

|  | Pre-Training (in inches) | Post-Training (in inches) | Mean Difference (in inches) | Improvement (%) |
|---|---|---|---|---|
| Wholebody Group ( N = 18 ) | 46.33 | 53.55 | 7.22 | 15.58 |
| Control Group ( N = 16 ) | 47.44 | 48.06 | 0.62 | 1.31 |

**SHOULDER FLEXION**

|  | Pre-Training (in inches) | Post-Training (in inches) | Mean Difference (in inches) | Improvement (%) |
|---|---|---|---|---|
| Wholebody Group ( N = 18 ) | 47.33 | 52.83 | 5.50 | 11.62 |
| Control Group ( N = 15 ) (a) | 50.75 | 51.25 | 0.50 | 0.99 |

**TRUNK FLEXION**

|  | Pre-Training (in inches) | Post-Training (in inches) | Mean Difference (in inches) | Improvement (%) |
|---|---|---|---|---|
| Wholebody Group ( N = 18 ) | 47.94 | 50.61 | 2.67 | 5.57 |
| Control Group ( N = 16 ) (a) | 50.50 | 50.63 | 0.13 | 0.26 |

a. One control group subject was omitted because of a shoulder injury.

Table 7-8. A comparison of the effects of training on the wholebody subject's level of lean muscle mass and body fat.

|  | Lean Body Mass (in lbs) | Body Fat (in lbs) | Fat (%) |
|---|---|---|---|
| Pre-Training ( N = 19 ) | 182.34 | 26.48 | 12.4 |
| Post-Training ( N = 19 ) | 180.48 | 27.50 | 13.0 |
| Mean Difference | - 1.86 | + 1.02 | 0.6 |

Table 7-9. Fat caliper measurements for subjects involved in "Project Total Conditioning." (a)

|  | Rochester (b) | | | USMA (c) | | |
|---|---|---|---|---|---|---|
|  | Pre-Training | Post-Training | Mean Difference | Pre-Training | Post-Training | Mean Difference |
| Wholebody Group ( N = 19 ) | 9.97 | 10.42 | +0.45 | 6.25 | 5.04 | - 1.21 |
| Control Group ( N = 10 ) | N.A. | N.A. | N.A. | 6.48 | 5.31 | - 1.17 |

a.  All measurements are in millimeters.

b.  The Rochester data is based on an average of five measurements: biceps, subcostal, umbilical, iliac, and subscapular.

c.  The USMA data is based on an average of several areas: chest, axilla, triceps, subscapular, abdomen, suprailliac, and frontal thigh.

Table 7-10. A comparison of the effects of a program using a Super Hip and Back Machine versus one using a DUOsymmetric POLYcontractile Hip and Back Machine.

VERTICAL JUMPING ABILITY

|  | Pre-Training (in inches) | Post-Training (in inches) | Mean Difference (in inches) | Improvement (%) |
|---|---|---|---|---|
| Regular Hip and Back | 22.222 | 22.722 | 0.50 | 2.25 |
| DUO - POLY Hip and Back | 21.45 | 22.86 | 1.41 | 6.57 |

of the 6 week study, the wholebody group (the prohibitive costs prevented the inclusion of the control group) was flown to Rochester, New York. At the University of Rochester Medical School, the relative level of lean body mass (muscle) and the body fat for each of the nineteen subjects was determined by means of the Whole Body Counter. By measuring the radiation given off by the potassium K in the body, the Whole Body Counter is able to provide an estimation of body fat. Table 8 presents the results.

Contrary to expectation, only eight out of nineteen subjects lowered the overall level of body fat. In fact, the group as a whole, averaged a slight increase in the amount of body fat. These calculations are in contradiction to both what might have been anticipated as the result of significant strength increases and to a visual interpolation of pre- and post-training photographs of the subjects (in only their gym shorts).*

A second source of anthropometric input was provided by fat-caliper measurements. Commonly referred to as skin-fold tests, these measurements are an accepted (although not entirely reliable) method of quantifying the relative amount of fat in the body. By measuring the thickness of specific areas of the body and comparing the change in thickness on a pre- post-treatment basis, the effect of the training on the body fat can be identified.

In "Project Total Conditioning," two sets of skin-fold measurements were obtained. In the first, the Rochester personnel provided fat caliper measurements of the nineteen wholebody group subjects. In the second set, USMA personnel measured both the wholebody and the control group members. Table 8 present the results.

Again the calculations are contradictory. The Rochester measurements showed a slight overall increase on the skin-fold tests, while the USMA calculations indicated a substantial decrease for both groups. On the USMA measurements, the wholebody group improved slightly better (19.4%) than did the control group (18.5%).

## THERMOGRAPHIC DIAGNOSIS

As an aside to the main areas of concern under investigation in "Project Total Conditioning," an effort was undertaken to evaluate the potential application of thermography to strength training. Basically, thermography is a procedure where skin temperature readings are

---

*Two possible sources of inaccuracy in the data are the 4% potential error inherent in the machine (as reported by the Rochester personnel) and the fact that the pre- and post-testing was conducted by two different sets of individuals.

visually obtained by means of a scanning camera and a display unit. In the past, thermography has been primarily concerned with various aspects of early breast cancer detection. Most thermographic instruments are still chiefly engaged in that application. However, the thermographic potential in medical diagnosis is apparently quite diverse and particularly promising in the field of orthopedics and peripheral circulation. Given that skin temperature recordings are representative of the circulatory situation in the examined tissues, the use of thermography may have many uses in the field of athletics.

In the present study, a consultant from AGA Corporation, the largest supplier of thermographic instruments in the world, was employed to visually record several workouts. At press time for this article, an analysis of his efforts and the implications of his findings has not been completed.

## CONCURRENT STUDIES

Two secondary studies were also conducted as part of "Project Total Conditioning." Lasting only four weeks, each investigative effort attempted to provide additional information concerning strength training practices and processes. In the first study twenty-four rugby team members participated in a project designed to examine the effects on overall neck strength of a twice weekly versus a three-times-a-week workout program. The content of the program (exercises, equipment, etc.) was the same as the one discussed in the section on neck strengthening. Somewhat surprisingly, the two-times-a-week program generated a slightly greater increase in neck strength (41.6%) than did the three-times-a-week (39.8%).

In the second project, twenty-two members of the USMA volleyball club team were involved in a study designed to determine the effect on their vertical jumping ability of an exercise program using the Nautilus Super Hip and Back Machine versus one which uses the Nautilus DUOsymmetric POLYcontractile Hip and Back Machine. Both programs consisted of each subject performing one set, three times weekly, on their appropriate machine. The total amount of expended time involved less than 60 seconds per workout. Table 10 presents the results of the training.

Although both programs increased the average vertical jumping ability of the subjects, the "DUO-POLY" workout—wherein the participant lowers the weight with one leg while being forced to keep the other leg in a contracted position—produced a greater increase. Since very little has been done regarding the study of the effects of "DUO-POLY" contractions on strength training results, this finding lends impetus to the need for additional investigative efforts.

## SUMMARY

In retrospect, considering the countless hours, the substantial cost, and the effort involved, the question might be asked: what was accomplished by "Project Total Conditioning"?

First and foremost, it was demonstrated that a strength training program, when properly conducted, **can** have a positive effect on the central components of physical fitness. In less than 6 weeks, high-intensity training of a relatively short duration increased the average overall strength of each subject by more than 58%. Neck strength was also significantly effected. The members of the wholebody and the neck-only group increased their aggregate level of neck strength by an average of 91.9% and 56.7% respectively. Contrary to most commonly held beliefs on the subject of strength training, the training also significantly improved the cardiovascular condition of the subjects. By maintaining the intensity of the workouts at a high level and by limiting the amount of rest between exercises, the training resulted in improvement on **each** of 60 separate measures of cardiovascular fitness. Contrary to widespread opinion, not only will a properly conducted program of strength training produce increases in muscular strength but will also significantly improve an individual's level of cardiovascular conditioning. The data suggests that some of these cardiovascular benefits apparently cannot be achieved by any other type of training. And finally, the experimental subjects increased their level of flexibility by an average of more than 10% on the three evaluative items.

In today's society, it is impossible to find any topic on which there is a shortage of rhetoric. Certainly, strength training is no exception. Unfortunately, much of this dialogue has been based on innuendo, superstition, and/or misinformation. This author feels that part of the misunderstanding has resulted from the fact that previous studies on the subject of conditioning have focused on only one or two aspects of the overall picture. For that reason many of the interrelationships of the effects of strength training have been either overlooked or misunderstood. "Project Total Conditioning" provides new insight and clarification into these interrelationships.

# CHAPTER 8
## Running

Robert Hoffman
Captain, Infantry

Why run?
How to run?
Basic training principles and considerations
Planning a program
Increasing speed
Measuring results
Equipment

## WHY RUN?

"Running is a total experience, that which some of us do best just as others find their satisfactions and fulfillment in skiing, mountain climbing, bicycling, snorkeling, pitching, or what have you. The experience is one that proceeds from one level to another. It can be merely physical fitness, or distraction, or religion. For some, sport is not a test but a therapy, not a trial but a reward, not a question, but an answer."

George Sheehan, MD*
(*from **Beginning Running,**
published by **Runner's
World Magazine,** 1972)

There are as many reasons for running as there are individuals who decide to run. The spectrum ranges from a desire to develop higher levels of physical fitness, to improving one's ability to perform in sports and athletics, to losing weight. Improvement in athletic performance may result from either increased speed or greater stamina (or both!).

## HOW TO RUN

In general, everyone has a natural gait—a way of running. For most individuals, little or no adjustment should be made in their natural gait. There are four basic components of this gait—foot plant, stride length, body carriage and aim movement.

Toni Nett (**Track Technique,** "Foot Plant in Running", March 1964) lists five guidelines for positioning the foot-fall when running.

1. Runners at all distances land first on the outside edge of the foot

and then roll inward. This has a shock-absorbing effect.

2. The precise point of contact along the outside edge of the foot varies with the speed of the runner.

3. In the 100- and 200-yard runs, the landing of the foot is high on the ball of the foot, near the joints of the little toe. In the 400, it is slightly farther back.

4. In the 800 and 1500, the contact point is the metatarsal arch area. The foot landing looks nearly flat.

5. In longer distances there is head-first contact. This involves landing on the heel and rolling on the balls of the feet during the stride. It is the most common method of running. It is easy on the legs and results in the **least** amount of muscle soreness.

Stride length, similar to foot-plant, also varies with the pace. It should be shortened as the athlete slows and stretched out as the speed increases. This component can obviously be affected by body type.

Body carriage will also vary with the pace. Sprinters will have a forward lean, with their center of gravity slightly forward of their foot-plant. This lean becomes less pronounced as distance increases and the pace slows. Distance runners should have an erect carriage, with their center of gravity directly above their foot-plant. This gives the distance runner maximum efficiency and power.

The arms should be carried comfortably at all speeds and distances. In general, your legs will move as fast as your arms. The hands should be loosely cupped, the elbow at about a 90° angle, and the arms should swing parallel to each other. Runners should avoid driving the arms across the body, attempting to keep all body movement going forward.

## BASIC TRAINING PRINCIPLES AND GUIDELINES
### STRESS

Running is a stress. The underlying principle of **all** conditioning is adapting to stress. Adaption refers to the fact that the body increases its resistance to stress through previous exposure to stress. Developed by Hans Selye and articulated into what is called a "general adaptation syndrome," this concept as applied to running means that an individual should run followed by a suitable recovery period for the adaptation to that stress to occur, followed by another stress and recovery, etc., gradually increasing the stress as the body's adaptation increases. If the athlete goes beyond his capacity to adapt, his body will incur some form of break-down, such as severe exhaustion. The secret of effective conditioning is determining proper doses of stress and recognizing the symptoms of over and under stressing.

## SPECIFICITY

An individual gets what he trains for—in other words, an individual's system adapts to the specific stresses it is given. An individual who walks becomes fit for walking. An individual who runs becomes fit for running.

## TRAINING EFFECT

Running can accomplish numerous individual improvements: increase the efficiency of the heart and the lungs, reduce body fat, tone and strengthen muscles and other connective tissue, and promote a feeling of health—both mental and physical. The training effect is usually observed in three main body systems: respiratory, cardiovascular, and muscular. The basic effects of running include:

1.  Respiratory System
    - Decreased breath rate.
    - Increased number of alveoli in lungs.
       (a) Increased vital capacity of lungs.
    - Increased effective exchange through the capillary net between alveoli and pulmonary artery and vein.
    - Increased endurance and efficiency of diaphragm and external intercostals.
2.  Cardiovascular System
    - Increased efficiency of heart,
       (a) Increased stroke volume.
       (b) Decreased resting pulse rate*
    - Increased capillarization of blood vessels.
       (a) Increased oxygen consumption.
    - Increased production of red blood cells.
       (a) Increased $O_2$ carrying capacity.
    - Increased coronary artery size. This gives the runner a greater chance to survive a heart attack, since the collateral circulation is greatly improved.
    - Increased thickness of artery walls, therefore increased strength of arteries.
    - Decreased blood pressure.

*The value of a lowered resting heart rate is that the heart, like any machine part, will last longer with less use. A resting heart rate of 55 beats per minute is not uncommon for a fairly well conditioned runner, while a heart rate of 75 beats per minute would be average for a poorly conditioned individual. In one day, this translates to 28,800 extra beats and in one year, 10,512,000 extra beats for the person with the higher heart rate!

3. Muscle System
   - Increased strength of muscle around bronchioles of lung.
   - Increased ability to store energy (glycogen) in muscles.
   - Increased ability of muscle to tolerate lactic acid buildup.
   - Increased efficiency of muscle to function for longer periods of time.
   - Increased efficiency of muscle to expel waste products of exercise (lactic acid).

## OXYGEN USE

The key to developing stamina is oxygen consumption. Running accomplishes two things: (1) the body is required to provide itself with large quantities of oxygen and (2) the system which carries the oxygen is tuned up. Endurance running—stamina training—is primarily an aerobic task. That is to say, it is an activity which requires that adequate oxygen be supplied to the muscles of the body **while** the exercise is being conducted. This is referred to as aerobic metabolism. For approximately the first 60 seconds of an all-out running effort, the aerobic as well as the anaerobic (non-oxygen requiring) metabolic systems are equally contributory. After the first 60 seconds, however, the aerobic system dominates. After this second period, the individual's ability to deliver oxygen to the working muscles is fundamental. (The reader is referred to Chapter 2 of this text for a more complete comparison between the aerobic and anaerobic systems.)

## HEART RATE

An individual is seldom equipped to make technically precise determinations of the physiological stress imposed upon his body during running. It is feasible, however, to determine post exercise pulse rates (first 10-20 seconds of recovery). The athlete should take his pulse for 10 seconds and multiply by six in order to obtain a reasonable accurate measure of his "running heart rate."

To achieve a training effect, a certain level of stress must be reached. The runner can approximate this level with the following calculations. First, compute the resting heart rate. Then run all out for approximately 60 seconds. Immediately take a pulse reading for 10 seconds, and multiply it by 6. This is an approximation of the individual's maximum heart rate. Next, take 75% of the difference between the resting heart rate and the maximum heart rate, and this add this to the resting heart rate.

The resulting heart rate is the level to be reached for a training effect. As fitness improves, the above calculations must be repeated to insure that intensity of workouts remains sufficient.

## REGULARITY

Conditioning can occur fairly quickly. Athletes can develop reasonably adequate levels of stamina within a matter of weeks. The reverse, however, is also true. Fitness vanishes relatively quickly when it is neglected. To gain and maintain stamina, an athlete should exercise at least every other day, with no long layoff periods during the year. Alternate day running is an application of the stress and adaptation principle. (Speed will be lost, more quickly than endurance.)

## STAGGERING

The individual runner should vary the distances he runs. He should mix his running program by performing a long run followed by a short easy run, followed by a day of rest, then a medium run, another short run, etc. Such a running program permits an adequate recovery time, provides a mental change of pace, and stimulates a reasonably fast opportunity for improvement. Based on the average of all average runs over a period of weeks and months, there are three general distances— short, average, and long. The average sets the boundaries. **Short** runs— for recovery and rest—should be about **half the daily average. Long** runs—used for consolidating an individual's weekly gains—should be about **twice the daily average.**

## PROGRESS

In theory, athletes can continue to gain stamina (endurance) indefinitely, so long as they increase their running in small increments which are within their limits of stress. Individual progress does not occur in a smooth upward curve. A plateau effect tends to occur, with a series of sudden improvements separated by stagnant periods. The athlete should be prepared to exercise through these stagnant periods. Athletes progress at their own rate. They establish their own starting points, their own standards of progress, and their own standards of success. For running programs, time, distance, and resting pulse rate are the best indicators of individual progress.

## PACING

Pacing refers to the speed an individual goes during a run. In a longitudinal sense, pacing also refers to the amount of stress (demand) that individuals place upon themselves over an extended period of time (week to week, month to month). In reference to pacing, athletes should remember one basic guideline: the greater the stress (pace), the less time the body can maintain the stress. Athletes should set their pace according to two factors: 1) the distance of the run and 2) the objectives of their running program.

A proper pace exists for every distance, relative to program objectives. In general, short runs are used for developing "speed" and require an "all-out effort" by the athlete. The pace for runs requiring more than 90 seconds should be relatively gentle. Gentle does **not** mean the slowest possible. Used primarily for building a **conditioning** base, moderate and long runs should be run at a pace which raises the individual's heart rate to approximately 140-150 beats per minute. Probably the most commonly used measure for determining whether or not an individual is running too fast on a conditioning run is the "talk test". If the athlete is gasping and can't talk during the run, he's going too fast.

## PLANNING A PROGRAM

### HOW TO START

The individual must have a goal for his program. It should be a sensible, feasible goal, such as developing stamina for a sport requiring aerobic endurance (e.g. basketball). Once the goal has been established, a plan for reaching that goal must be developed. The three key ingredients of this plan must be **intensity, duration,** and **frequency.** As mentioned earlier, a certain level of stress must be reached in order to achieve a training effect. The runner can thus use heart rate as a means of gauging the intensity of his workouts. This method also permits increasing the intensity as conditioning increases.

Most experts agree that it takes at least ten minutes of running at the above mentioned intensity to achieve a desired training effect. This is a good starting point. If the individual cannot run the entire ten minutes, then run and walk, or even just walk. The duration of runs can be increased as the level of conditioning improves.

The frequency of workouts should be at least every other day to begin with. Running must become a habit if the individual is to become fit. However, even as the level of conditioning improves, the runner should probably not run more than six days a week, allowing the body one day of rest.

By considerating intensity, duration, and frequency, the runner can most efficiently build a base of conditioning. A typical starting program might be:

### 1st Week
Monday-Wednesday-Friday-Sunday/15-20 min.
Tuesday-Thursday-Saturday—Rest

### 2nd Week
Monday/20-25 min.
Wednesday-Friday-Sunday/15-20 min.
Tuesday-Thursday-Saturday/Rest

### 3rd Week
Monday-Wednesday/20-25 min.
Friday-Sunday/15-20 min.
Tuesday-Thursday-Saturday/Rest

### 4th Week
Monday-Wednesday-Friday/20-25 min.
Sunday/25-30 min.
Tuesday-Thursday-Saturday/Rest

Within ten weeks at a gradual level of progression, an athlete should be able to lengthen the amount of time spent on at least one weekly run to 40-45 minutes while still providing for an adequate amount of rest. The main point to be considered is that an individual should establish a conditioning base **before** he undertakes a prolonged run.

## IMPROVING THE 2 MILE RUN TIME

For individuals who wish to improve their time in running a moderate (or greater) distance, such as the 2 mile run, a program employing varying distances of short, medium, and long runs is recommended. (Editor's Note: The 2 mile run is an integral item in both the USMA and the U.S. Army physical ability testing programs.)

Individuals who are somewhat below average in their level of personal fitness should begin with a program of approximately 10 miles per week. An example of such as program would be:

| DAY | LENGTH | DISTANCE RUN |
|---|---|---|
| Monday | Medium | 15% - 1.5 miles |
| Tuesday | Medium or Short | 10% - 1.0 mile |
| Wednesday | Long | 20% - 2.0 miles |
| Thursday | Short | 5% - .5 mile |
| Friday | Medium | 15% - 1.5 miles |
| Saturday | Long | 30% - 3.0 miles |
| Sunday | Short or Rest | 5% - .5 mile |
| | | 10.0 miles |

- The weekly load should be increased at the following rate:
    Short Runs - not increased in length
    Medium Runs - increased in length by 1 mile every 2 or 3 weeks
    Long Runs - increased by 1 mile each week
  - Individuals should not start with a mileage which is too great, because they will not be able to tolerate the subsequent increased load required by schedule without possibly breaking down physically. After **12 weeks,** an individual will have increased his training load considerably to a point where his schedule should read approximately as follows:

| DAY | LENGTH | DISTANCE |
|---|---|---|
| Monday | Medium | 3 miles |
| Tuesday | Medium/Short | 2.5 miles |
| Wednesday | Long | 5 miles |
| Thursday | Short | 2 miles |
| Friday | Medium | 3 miles |
| Saturday | Long | 7.5 miles |
| Sunday | Short/Rest | 2 miles |
| | | 25 miles |

  - About 7 weeks before the 2 mile event, the runner should begin to sharpen (improve speed) so that his 2 mile time might be lowered substantially.
  - Although the weekly schedule should continue to total essentially the same amount of mileage per week, the overall workout requirement should be modified to include speed workouts. For example, the following program might be employed:

| DAY | EFFORT |
|---|---|
| Monday | Short run |
| Tuesday | Speed work |
| Wednesday | Long run |
| Thursday | Speed work |
| Friday | Speed work |
| Saturday | Medium run |
| Sunday | Rest |

SPEED WORKOUTS

Speed workouts (as the name implies) are runs which are designed to improve the speed at which a distance can be run. Run at either an almost all-out effort or a maximum pace, speed workouts permit an individual to stress himself at varying distances. The ultimate goal is to be able to run a proposed distance (e.g. 2 miles) at a **maximum** pace.

To improve 2 mile run time, the initial speed workouts should be interval 880 yd and 440 yd runs with 3 to 4 minutes rest between each interval. The effort should be at faster-than-planned pace for the 2 mile run. On each day where a speed effort is planned, the interval indicated below is recommended:

| WEEK | DISTANCE |
|------|----------|
| 1st Week | 3 x 880 yds |
| 2nd Week | 3 x 880 yds, 1 x 440 yds |
| 3rd Week | 4 x 880 yds |
| 4th Week | 4 x 880 yds, 1 x 440 yds |
| 5th Week | 5 x 880 yds |
| 6th Week | 5 x 880 yds, 1 x 440 yds |
| 7th Week | 5 x 880 yds or 3 one mile runs |

After about 4 weeks, one of the speed workouts each week should be replaced with a 2-3 mile run at race pace. In addition, one more speed workout may be replaced by a 2 mile run using fast-slow 50 yd sprints. Fast-slow sprints are runs which alternate all-out sprints with gentle jogging for approximately equal distances. Such workouts should tremendously improve the runner's speed in a very short time.

INCREASING SPEED

Basic speed can be improved by increasing flexibility and by increasing strength in the related muscle groups. An increase in flexibility results in an increase in the range of muscle movement about the joint. The obvious result is an increase in stride length. An athlete who puts this theory into practice, can increase his stride by approximately two inches. In a forty-yard dash, this increase in stride would amount to thirty-four inches or almost three feet over this distance.

It is important to note that the fastest 100-yard dash runner is the individual who can maintain his speed for the full distance. The relationship of strength to speed is essential. Strength in running is defined as the ability to maintain speed for a long period of time.

Most athletes are aware of the basic mechanics of running, such as the alignment of the head, hips and knees, body angle, and foot placement. However, it is strongly recommended by many sprint coaches that the arms be used to direct the proper leg action.

To improve running mechanics, the first thing to work on is the arm swing. A 90-degree angle at the elbow produces a short pendulum, and allows the arm to swing quickly and powerfully. This short arm movement produces short, fast movements in the legs. It is essential to get the arms swinging straight ahead. This keeps the center of gravity moving in the desired path. The arms should never swing across the body because other motions are introduced into the action which will reduce speed.

Directly related to the arm swing is the correct arm position which is achieved by controlling the elbows with the hands. The elbows must pass close to the hips for maximum efficiency. On the backward swing, the arm is brought to a point where, if an individual dropped his hand directly down, it would fall in his back pocket. On the forward swing, bring the hand to a point at the collar bone level. If he brings it any higher, he will raise the center of gravity, thereby reducing his speed.

Throughout the years coaches have looked for various ways to improve the speed of their runners. Running with weights, running up stadium stairs, and running through water have all been tried with varying degrees of success. In 1960, an Australian named Cecil Hensley startled the running world when he announced that he had been using cars to tow his runners. He claimed that the rapid improvement of his runners was due to this method. The theory was that this would teach the legs to move faster. This method of training is difficult at best, not to mention the dangers involved. More recently Frank Costello of the University of Maryland has developed a theory based upon downhill running. Once a certain level of conditioning has been reached, this program involves three speed workouts a week. A moderate downhill stretch of about 60 yards is required, ideally grassy with no rocks, holes or other dangerous features. Workouts consist of eight 40-yard dashes at top speed learning to move the arms and legs fast enough to maintain balance. Costello reports drastic improvements in the speed of his runners using this technique.

## MEASURING SUCCESS

For the athlete, the major goal of a running program is whether or not it results either directly or indirectly in personal improvement in his ability to perform in his sport. There are, however, at least three other major criteria by which a running program can be evaluated: ability to run a specific distance at a predetermined pace, individual body weight, and individual pulse rate. In order to identify improvement, a record of pertinent information concerning the running program should be kept. On a daily basis, the following information should be recorded:

(1) Distance, route, and time of the run
(2) Bodyweight (should be taken under similar conditions every

day—**same** time, same clothing, etc.)

(3) Pulse rate (should be taken under similar conditions every day—either wrist or neck pulse, same time, resting conditions, etc.)

(4) Unusual factors (aches and pains, external mitigating factors, amount of sleep, mental state, etc.)

To determine an individual's level of performance at the start of a running program, Cooper's 12 minute walk/run can be repeated periodically to measure progress.

EQUIPMENT

A. **Clothing.** Participation in a running program requires little equipment. A shirt, pants, socks and shoes are the basic uniform. A white or light colored shirt that will reflect the sun's rays is usually worn on warm, or hot clear days. In cooler weather, heavier shirts with long sleeves are worn. The colder it gets, the more clothes are worn. In very cold weather, wear thermal underwear, tops and bottoms, nylon running pants, mittens (or socks over the hands), a wool hat, and a windbreaker. Zippers, hoods, and pockets for gloves and hats are desirable items for adjusting to changing temperatures.

B. **Shoes.** There are several important considerations in choosing a running shoe:

1. **The needs of the individual.** In general, the individual will choose a training shoe over a racing shoe. As distance increases, more protection is needed for the foot. Each foot strikes the ground approximately 5000 times during a one hour run. Good shoes are important in the prevention of foot and leg injuries.

2. **Weight.** Lightness is important only up to a point. Again, as distance increases, you need extra protection. Thicker soles became a more desirable feature. Statistics have shown that leg and foot injuries are more prevalent in runners who weigh more than 170 pounds.

3. **Comfort.** The sole must serve a dual purpose. It must be comfortable and yet absorb shock. Simple sponge rubber is too soft. It should be flexible from the balls of the feet forward. Yet there should be limited flexibility from that point to the rear of the shoe.

The upper should be snug, but not overly tight. Both nylon and leather have their advantages. Nowadays shoes are already broken in, so how they feel in the store should be how they feel when running in them.

4. **Heel.** Shoe producers have made great changes in heel construction in recent years. They have widened the heel to prevent instability, and have raised the heel slightly higher than the ball of the foot.

5. **Arch.** The arch support is a very individual item. Some runners

need it and others don't. If it feels uncomfortable, rip it out.

6. **Last.** This is the shape of the bottom of the shoe. Trace it on paper, and stand on the tracing with bare feet. It any part of the foot extends outside of the tracing, the runner will most likely suffer twisting, cramping or slipping.

7. **Price.** An individual who runs 5 days a week can expect to go through an average of two pairs of shoes a year. That's $30-$50 at today's prices for name brand running shoes. Competition among shoe manufacturers may lower prices somewhat in the future. What about bargain priced shoes? At first glance, these shoes are often indistinguishable from the name brand shoes that they are trying to imitate. **Runner's World** magazine lists several items to check before buying these cheaper shoes. First the sole. Often it will not bend at all, or if it does, it will only bend in the middle of the shoe. The most flexible part should be forward of the ball of the foot, which is where the foot bends during running. The sole material is often porous, and will wear quickly. These manufacturers often save by using poor quality insoles, which disintegrate in the presence of sweat. The heel cup likewise is of poor quality.

While some runners claim that their bargain shoes are as good as the name brands; in general you get what you pay for. In this case it may be blisters, shin splints, etc.


## MISCELLANEOUS

All runners have experienced one, if not all, of the following phenomena associated with running. None of them have been conclusively explained by science, but there are generally accepted theories concerning each of them.

**Muscle soreness** — This problem will beset everyone either upon beginning a running program, or upon returning to one after a long layoff. The pain is probably due to actual injury of the muscle, usually at its attachment to the tendon. Secondly, histamine, lactic acid, and other substances are produced, causing edema and pain. Symptoms usually appear after about 12 hours, become more severe the next day, and fade away within 4-6 days. Light exercise will promote faster recovery. The repair of the damaged tissue results in a stronger muscle, less susceptible to further injuries.

**Side aches** — Initially, respiratory muscles are working anaerobically. When the system changes over to aerobic there is a time lag in the redistribution of the blood, with not enough $O_2$ going to the diaphragm. This is most common in untrained persons or after a meal. A possible solution is to pick up the pace, forcing the system to reach maximum

$O_2$ utilization faster. Another possibility is to hold the breath.

**Second wind** — It is generally agreed that this condition occurs when a "steady state" is reached. That is, when the $O_2$ brought in is equal to the requirements created by the exercise. This may occur at the switch over from the anaerobic to aerobic energy production.

**Mental Staleness** — Many runners begin to notice negative results from continuous workouts. Coaches have felt that runners "burn out" from going all out for long periods of time. Even for the casual runner this can be a problem. Missing a workout is not the end of the world. However, runners must be cautioned not to allow themselves to fall prey to using staleness as an excuse for laziness.

**Eating & Drinking Before Running** — For the competitive runner, eating before a race can cause a lowered performance. Blood that could carry $O_2$ to the functioning muscles may be diverted to the muscles of digestion. Eating before running should not be a significant problem for the casual runner. The feeling of discomfort associated with food in the gut may be reason enough for some not to eat before running. It is mostly psychological, however. Likewise for drinking. In fact, on a hot, humid day it may be essential to drink a glass of water before going on a long run. The body's fluids must be maintained. After running, the individual should drink until he is no longer thirsty, then drink a little more. This is a good guideline for replacing the body's fluids.

**Fasting** — Lately this practice has become popular among marathoners. While most agree that lowered body weight is an important plus for the long distance runner, they are testing a relatively new theory. That is that by fasting during training, they can train their bodies to burn fats along with carbohydrates. Fats produce more energy per gram, and are usually not burned except in the absence of carbohydrates. Theoretically, these runners will be able to burn fats and carbohydrates throughout the 26.2 miles of a marathon.

---

As mentioned in the introduction, while there is currently no hard proof for any of these theories, there is agreement that these are plausible explanations.

---

# CHAPTER 9
## Women and Athletics

James A. Peterson, Ph.D.
and
Susan L. Peterson
Director of Self-Defense for Women

Physiological differences
Mythology of women and sport
Female does not mean inferior

Despite the fact that women comprise more than one-half of the population of the United States, relatively little accurate information exists concerning their true potential for performing in sports and athletics. Although a review of the literature suggests that men have traditionally demonstrated greater levels of physical prowess than women, a wide variety of reasons (e.g. cultural, motivational, physiological) have been advanced to explain the disparity of performance between men and women. On one hand, many individuals claim that women simply are so genetically different than men that except for a few isolated cases of olympic-caliber participants, women will never be able to perform at an "adequate level." On the other hand, other individuals state that the performance disparity between men and women is entirely the result of cultural biases. Society in its attempts to direct young girls to predetermined roles simply does not provide the average young women with the opportunity to play and develop athletically.

In actuality, the truth lies somewhere between the two aforementioned polarities. While there is validity in the claim that physiological differences exist between men and women, there is **no doubt** that women have been shortchanged in the athletic arena. Unfortunately, until which time that additional research is undertaken to scientifically assess the physical capabilities of women, the actual physical potential of women will essentially remain a matter of conjecture and debate.

## PHYSIOLOGICAL DIFFERENCES

A review of the literature relating to physiological differences between men and women suggests that several genetic differences exist. In the interest of lending clarity and order to a discussion of these differences, four comparative areas can be examined: anthropometrics, body composition, cardiorespiratory factors, and menstruation. All data, unless otherwise noted, represents the "mean average" for the group under discussion. In addition, while a substantial amount of information could be collected which could examine the genetic similarities between men and women, only differences between the two sexes are discussed in this chapter.

## ANTHROPOMETRIC AND BODY COMPOSITION FACTORS

A summary of adult male and female anthropometric and body composition comparisons is presented in Table 9-1. The implications of the existing differences on physical performance are significant. The female possesses only about half the amount of lean muscle mass (LMM) than does the male. As a result of this greater quantity of LMM and coupled with their greater size and level of strength, men generally perform far better than women in activities which require explosive power; e.g. sprinting, basketball throw, medicine ball put, and jumping events. Even when size is held constant, however, females are only 80% as strong as males. Researchers attribute this condition to hormonal changes (the production of testosterone) which occur in males at puberty. On the other hand, numerous studies on women's strength have indicated that in this country, women generally reach their peak performance at about the age of 12½ or one year before menstruation begins. It is hypothesized that the lack of testosterone, coupled with the addition of estrogen—a hormone believed to inhibit the development of muscle mass, causes the "performance slowdown" in women.

The elbow joint is another anthropometric characteristic on which men and women frequently differ. While a few researchers have taken exception to the conclusion that these differences in the elbow joint can affect athletic performance, many investigators have stated otherwise. These individuals found that when the female elbow joint is hyperextended and the arms are extended in a supinated position, the elbows are much closer to each other than in males, and the female arms form an "X" whereas the male arms form parallel lines extending from the shoulders. These researchers speculate that this angular displacement of the female forearm to the upper arm results in poorer performances in the throwing activities such as discus and javelin events, and is a handicap in sports requiring maximum leverage, such as tennis and gymnastics.

Another physiological difference is the angle of the femur with the pelvis. A women's pelvis is ½" wider and is rounder than the man's. From the slightly wider pelvis, the femurs extend at a greater angle. Some researchers speculate that the X-shaped leg tendencies, the joint distensions, and the softer joints and ligaments in the pelvic girdle of women are disadvantageous in running and jumping events.

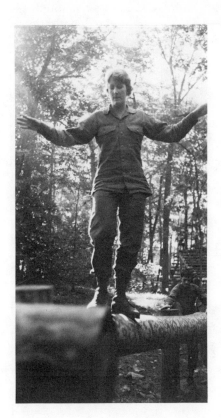

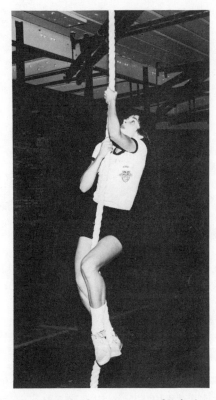

Women at West Point: documentation that **female does not equal inferior.**

Table 9-1. A Summary of Anthropometric and Body Composition Comparisons Between Men and Women

| Anthropometric & Body Composition Characteristic | Physical Performance Advantage | MAN | WOMAN | Physical Performance Advantage |
|---|---|---|---|---|
| Height* | greater lung volume, speed, power | taller | shorter | quick rotary movements |
| Weight* | throwing power | 20-25% heavier | | |
| Muscle Mass % of Total Body Weight | power, speed, strength | ( 50%) greater | | |
| Body Fat % of Total Body Weight | | | (20-30%) greater | buoyancy |
| Center of Gravity | rotary movement | higher | lower | balance |
| Pelvis | running speed | shallower, narrower, heavier | wider, rounder | lateral swag in running |
| Hips | power production | narrower | wider | stability |
| Chest Girth | ventilation capacity | greater | | |
| Leg Length | acceleration, speed, power, greater kicking velocity | longer | shorter | agility |
| Elbow Joint | leverage in throwing | arms parallel from shoulders | arms form an "X" from the shoulders | |

*According to the US Public Health Service, the average 18 year old male is 70.2″ tall and weighs 144.8 lbs. The average 18 year old female is 64.4″ tall and weighs 126.2 lbs. (Source 1975 World Almanac).

In terms of body composition, women have less bone mass, less muscle component, but more fat than men. This combination of more fat and less muscle per unit volume has a negative effect upon physical performances requiring strength, speed, and power. In addition, women accumulate fat on the waist, arms, and thighs, whereas men accumulate fat primarily on the back, chest, and abdomen. This differential distribution effects movement efficiency. Since women have a relatively longer trunk and shorter legs, their weight is distributed lower than it is in the males. The pelvis and thighs of women contain a greater amount of weight. Thus, the female center of gravity is 6% lower than that of the males. The greater weight in the thigh in proportion to the muscle mass provides the female lower limbs with more inertia and more resistance to rotary movement than the lower limbs of men. As a result, on a proportional muscular force basis, the speed of movement in females is slower.

## CARDIORESPIRATORY FACTORS

Physical activity involving large muscle groups requires that the body undergo certain physiological changes. The body must provide the energy for muscular contraction either aerobically, as in the distance events when oxygen is provided in amounts as needed, or anaerobically, as in sprinting, when short periods of gross muscle contraction are made in excess of available oxygen.

The physiological mechanisms that influence both aerobic and anaerobic work, and consequently greatly effect sports performance, have been extensively investigated. The studies in this area have primarily focused on the efficiency of the oxygen absorption system, efficiency of the oxygen transport system, and the ability of the body to tolerate accumulated fatigue products. Because the circulatory and the respiratory systems are the cardinal limiting factors in these matters, it is necessary to examine the potential effect of cardiorespiratory differences between men and women on physical performance.

Table 9-2 presents a comparative summary of adult male and female cardiorespiratory factors. Several differences exist, most of which place a woman at a disadvantage if she is to be compared to a man in endurance activities. Collectively summarized, the differences that are important in terms of physical performance are cardiovascular characteristics, aerobic activity, blood characteristics, and heat tolerance. The implication of these differences are twofold: (1) men have a greater potential for endurance that cannot by matched by women; and (2) at sub-maximal work levels, women have to work much harder to accomplish the same amount of work.

Table 9-2. A Summary of Cardiorespiratory Comparisons Between Men and Women

| Cardiorespiratory Component | | Physical Performance Advantage |
| --- | --- | --- |
| Heart Volume | greater ( $>$ 25%) | (1) Men have a greater potential for endurance that apparently cannot be matched by women. |
| Red Blood Cells | greater ( $>$ 8%) | |
| Hemoglobin | greater ( $>$ 10-15%) | |
| Vital Capacity | greater ( $>$ 25-30%) | |
| Cardiac Output | greater ( $>$ 10%) | (2) At submaximal work levels, women have to work much harder than men to accomplish the same amount of work. |
| Maximum Heart Rate | greater ( $>$ 2-4%) | |
| $VO_2MAX$ | greater ( $>$ 15-35%) | |
| Diffusing capacity of alveolar membrane | greater ( $>$ 10%) | |

There are several cardiovascular differences which can be attributed to gender. Physically, the male heart and lungs are larger than those of the female. Not only are they larger, but the relative weight of a man's heart and lungs to his total body weight is greater. The larger male heart and lungs produce higher stroke volumes (the amount of blood forced from the heart for each beat) and vital capacities (maximum volume of air that can be expelled from the lungs following a maximum inspiration) than those of women. In addition, the heart rate of men is approximately 5 to 8 beats/min slower than that of women, both at rest and at all levels of exercise. Another cardiovascular difference concerns the oxygen content in arterial blood. Due to higher hemoglobin values, men have more oxygen in their arterial blood than do women. Accordingly, the variations of oxygen content of arterial blood that occur during exercise are met by compensatory changes in cardiac output. Since maximal cardiac output is limited somewhat by the size of the heart, the female cannot (comparatively) internally adjust for the lower content of oxygen in the arterial blood. As a result, women can consume less oxygen than men.

The second cardiorespiratory factor affected by these differences is aerobic capacity. This factor is important because it is an indication of the ability of an individual to continue delivering the required amount of oxygen demanded by the working muscles under varying work loads. Aerobic capacity is generally expressed as oxygen uptake, ($VO_2$), which is defined as the volume of oxygen that can be extracted from the inspired air. Maximum oxygen uptake ($VO_2max$) is the maximum amount of oxygen that can be extracted while performing strenuous work and is expressed as liters per minute. Once individuals reach their $VO_2max$, work may be continued until the building of waste products forces a cessation of the work. Numerous researchers have found that on a $VO_2max$ test (a measure generally considered to be the best single criterion of cardiovascular endurance), men are superior to women.

The third cardiorespiratory component affected by differences between men and women concerns blood characteristics. Men have a higher percentage of red blood cells, the oxygen-carrying component in the body. Men also have a 30% greater amount of total body hemoglobin, due to their greater body size. The lower average hemoglobin content of arterial blood in women has frequently been advanced by researchers as a principal explanation for the lower aerobic capacity of women. During heavy exercise women have to increase cardiac output in order to compensate for lower arterial oxygen hemoglobin. During vigorous physical exertion, women have to increase their heart rate since stroke volume and performance are limited by total blood volume. Accordingly, for a given sub-maximal work load, since women are always operating at a level closer to their maximum than men, they will reach exhaustion sooner.

The fourth cardiorespiratory factor to be examined is heat tolerance. Since heat is a limiting factor in physical performance, both men and women must develop methods of handling temperature increases. There are two types of heat. Metabolic heat is an index of the higher internal body temperatures which are generated by an individual's physical activity. Ambient heat is the measure of environmental temperature. It interacts with humidity to produce thermal stresses on the body. Researchers have found that women have a higher body temperature at rest than men, fewer sweat glands, lower sweat production, and a propensity to start sweating at higher temperatures than do men. A woman's greater amount of adipose tissue serves as insulation and inhibits heat dissipation. These differences have an important implication for physical performance. Women have less tolerance to heat than men. As a result, women are more subject to heat stress than men. Under heat conditions at all levels of work, a woman's heart rate is substantially faster than that of a man's. Accordingly, under higher levels of heat condition, a woman has to work much harder than a man to perform similar work loads.

## MENSTRUATION FACTORS

Answer to questions relating to the effect of the menstrual cycle on physical performance remain largely a matter of educated speculation. Such questions are very difficult to answer experimentally, due to the extreme variability of subjects' menstrual phases. Much of the existing information on the subject has been provided by physicians. The reliability of instruments commonly used to obtain such data (self-report inventories or questionnaire) has never been validated. In addition, experimental bias and the Hawthorne effect (subject knows she is a participant in a study, thereby affecting her perceptions and her performances) may have influenced such data.

The literature is somewhat more clear with regard to whether or not women should be restricted from physical participation during menstruation. The majority of recent investigations on this question expresses the opinion that sports activity has **little effect** on menstruation and that **no restriction** should be placed on the physical activity of average women at any phase of their cycle. At the present time, little is known about the influence of "psychological effects" on physical activity during the menstrual cycle.

## MYTHOLOGY OF WOMEN AND SPORT

A considerable amount of mythology exists concerning whether or not women should participate in sports and athletics. Based on unfounded claims and misinformation, such mythology has long served as a foundation to support the premise that sport and athletics should be a **male** domain. Title IX (federal legislation which mandates equitable funds and facilities for women's athletic programs), changing societal mores, and an enlightened populace are gradually debunking such nonsense. Six of the more traditional myths concerning women's sports participation are discussed in this section.

*MYTH #1. Exercise in unladylike.*

The old adage that men sweat, women perspire, and ladies glow is merely a way of restating predetermined *roles* for women. Exercise is no more the perview of manhood than cooking is for women.

*Myth #2. Vigorous activity might harm a woman's reproductive organs or cause menstrual problems.*

On the contrary, physical activity generally improves menses for most women. No scientific evidence exists which has proven that physical activity has a detrimental effect on menses.

*Myth #3. Women cannot reach peak performance during menstruation.*

On the contrary, many national and international track records were broken by women at *all* stages of menses. In fact, one olympic record was broken while the performer was pregnant. In addition, some evidence exists which suggests that a woman's athletic performance actually improves after childbirth.

*Myth #4. Women should avoid contact sports because of possible breast damage.*

No medical evidence exists to support such a claim. In fact, male athletes may have more cause for concern arising from the relatively unprotected nature of the male genitals.

*Myth #5. Women will develop bulging muscles.*

Although women generally have not been given the opportunity to "exercise too much," both the existing research and pragmatic observations of selected situations (e.g. women at West Point) suggest that this myth has no validity. Frankly, most women do not have the hormonal capability of developing "bulging" muscles. Women can increase their strength, however, by means of properly organized muscular development programs (see Chapter 3-6).

*Myth #6. Women are more likely to be injured in sports than men.*

The American Medical Association's committee on sports emphatically disagrees with such a conclusion. There is no genetic reason for women to be more susceptible to athletic injuries than men. Women athletes (in this author's opinion) should be aware, however, that for vigorous sports (e.g. basketball), it is essential that an adequate conditioning base be developed before extensive physical stress is undertaken. Many women athletes suffer from various lower limb medical discomforts (e.g. shin splints, stress fractures, etc.) simply because a proper conditioning base is not laid before the demands on their bodies become too great.

## FEMALE DOES NOT EQUAL INFERIOR

Given the rapid growth of athletic programs for women at all educational levels and the marked improvment in general sports performance by women athletes, it is relatively easy to surmise that women have not begun to reach their physical potential. In fact, current physiological data on women may provide only a superficial description of the "emerging" women athlete. In years to come as the opportunities for athletic participation by women continue to expand, let no one doubt that *female does not equal inferior!*

# CHAPTER 10
## Nutrition and Athletics

James A. Peterson, Ph.D.

Physiology of nutrition
Energy expenditure in exercise
The pre-game meal
How much protein is enough?
Carbohydrate loading
The hazards of starvation
Dietary supplements
Weight loss
Weight gain

Athletes frequently spend untold hours developing and practicing their sport skills. Similarly, coaches often drill their teams to the utmost limits of their physical capabilities. Sportsmen everywhere literally devour every available piece of literature on their activity. Despite such enthusiasm and sincerity, the same individuals virtually ignore the proper principles of nutrition.

Nothing is more indicative of the regressive thinking surrounding nutrition than the traditional pre-game meal of steak, baked potato, green peas, toast, fruit cup, and sweetened tea three to four hours before game time. On the contrary, the American Medical Association points out that the athlete's protein supplies are established at least 48 hours prior to game time. As a result, when an athlete consumes more than enough protein, no benefit to physical performance is achieved. Unfortunately, coaches and athletes who believe otherwise about the value of "steak therapy" are not easily deterred.

### PHYSIOLOGY OF NUTRITION

In order to better understand how adherence to proper nutrition principles can improve athletic performance, it is beneficial to examine certain basic facts about how the body functions. In general, there are several factors to be considered:

(1) In order for the human body to function, it needs energy.

(2) The "fuel" the body uses to obtain energy is provided by the food the individual consumes.

(3) When oxygen is supplied to this fuel, it burns giving off energy.

(4) In the human body, oxygen (supplied by the blood stream) helps the body burn the fuel to supply energy.

(5) Every food contains substances (referred to as **nutrients**) which

supply body building ingredients. **No** one food has all the nutrients in it that the body requires. Since every nutrient has a specific use in the body, a **combination** of nutrients are needed for a well balanced diet. The actual nutrient needs vary from individual to individual. Table 10-1 lists the six nutrients and a brief description of the function of each.

(6) A calorie is the unit used to measure the "fuel value" of food. A gram of fats has more than twice the calories (9) than a gram of either protein or carbohydrates (4 each).

(7) The proper timing of meals is very important for the athlete. The AMA's Medical Aspects of Sports Committee states that for the normal schedule of digestion, it usually takes 2 to 4 hours for a meal to traverse the digestive system of the stomach. In another two hours, it will pass through the small intestine. Emotional tension, however, may slow the process.


ENERGY EXPENDITURE IN EXERCISE

The average adult man will burn up 2400 to 4500 calories a day depending upon his size, metabolic rate, and the amount and kind of exercise he gets. Active individuals, on the other hand, can consume up to 6000 calories a day and not gain weight.

The cost in calories of different types of exercise has been established and is illustrated in Table 10-2. The number of calories expended depends on how strenuously these activities are undertaken. For example, canoeing upstream in fast water will use up more than the 230 calories per hour, as specified in the Table 10-2—and jogging at a gentle pace will obviously use up less than jogging at a faster pace.

The figures on energy expenditure through various activities are probably underestimated. They are usually derived by measuring the amount of oxygen consumed during a specific bout of exercise and then computing the equivalent number of calories burned. However, the effects of exercise continue after the actual time in which the exercise is performed. Body processes have been stepped-up and only gradually are lowered; this takes energy—sometimes for long periods after the exercise is stopped.

Energy expended is also affected by body weight since in those activities where the individual has to move his own weight, energy costs are increased for the heavier person and decreased for the lighter individual. To illustrate, a person walking 3 mph, weighing 100 pounds, will burn as few as 50 calories in 15 minutes, while someone weighing 200 pounds would use up as many as 80 calories in the same length of time. The athlete should remember that although it takes an hour's jogging to use

## Table 10-1. The six basic nutrients.

**PROTEIN**

Proteins are the fundamental structural element of every cell of the body. Its name is derived from a Greek word meaning "of first importance." Proteins are composed of carbon, hydrogen, oxygen, nitrogen and sulfur. Protein is necessary to build and repair body tissue but some proteins are better than others for these purposes: A complete protein contains the essential amino acids in the most useful proportions and will best build and repair tissue. The best proportioned proteins are found in such foods as meat, fish, cheese, eggs, poultry, and milk. Plant proteins are not as complete — these are found in grains, legumes, (such as beans, peas) and nuts and need balancing with animal proteins to supply the body with usable protein elements.

**CARBOHYDRATE**

Carbohydrate foods are the major sources of calories for people all over the world. They make up 50 to 60% of the American diet and in other countries the percentage is even higher. They are easily digested and constitute the cheapest form of food energy. They are composed of carbon, hydrogen, and oxygen and exist as complex sugars and starches which are converted, through digestion, to simpler sugars which the body can utilize for energy. Carbohydrates include cellulose which is important as roughage in the digestive tract. All carbohydrate eventually becomes glucose, a simple sugar which travels through the blood stream and serves as a source of energy for the body tissues. Important carbohydrates are sugars, starches, syrups, and honey and are major constituents of vegetables, fruits, breads and cereals.

**FATS**

Fats are compounds of fatty acids and glycerol — another complex structure of carbon, hydrogen and oxygen — insoluble in water and greasy to the touch. The different fats in each food help give the food its particular flavor and texture. Fats are especially important because they produce more concentrated energy, almost 2½ times as much as either proteins or carbohydrates. They have a high satiety value — because they take longer to digest than other nutrients they keep us from feeling hungry for longer periods of time. Fats also are carriers of the fat soluble vitamins — A, D, E and K. They can be generally classified as animal fats and vegetable fats — the former found in meats, eggs, milk, butter — the latter in margarine, vegetable oils, mayonnaise, and salad dressing.

**MINERALS**

Minerals are found in foods mixed or combined with proteins, fats and carbohydrates. Calcium and phosphorus are minerals which give rigidity to the bones and teeth. Milk is a good source of both. Minerals are also needed for normal blood clotting and proper functioning of the nervous system. Iron is a mineral, essential in the diet since lack of it can produce anemia and make us feel tired and listless. Meat and enriched bread are good sources of iron. Other minerals are essential to help maintain a normal acid-base balance in the body and other important functions.

**VITAMINS**

Vitamins are complex organic compounds which are found in foodstuffs. They perform specific vital functions in the cells and tissues of the body. They are called accessory food factors and are needed for normal health which includes good eyesight, strong teeth and bones, freedom from infection and disease, normal functioning of the nervous system, tissue respiration and other functions.

**WATER**

Water is also essential to life. It is a necessary constituent of digestive juices and of every cell and tissue of the body. Two-thirds of the body weight is water. It is a major component of blood, lymph and other secretions of the body, and helps regulate body temperature. As a carrier, it aids digestion, absorption, circulation, and excretion. Moisture is necessary for the functioning of every organ of the body. Most foods contain a large percentage of water.

Table 10-2. Energy expenditure by a 150 pound person in various activities*

| Activity | Gross Energy Cost-Cal per hr. |
|---|---|
| **A. Rest and Light Activity** | **50-200** |
| Lying down or sleeping | 80 |
| Sitting | 100 |
| Driving an automobile | 120 |
| Standing | 140 |
| **B. Moderate Activity** | **200-350** |
| Bicycling (5½ mph) | 210 |
| Walking (2½ mph) | 210 |
| Canoeing (2½ mph) | 230 |
| Golf | 250 |
| Bowling | 270 |
| Fencing | 300 |
| Rowboating (2½ mph) | 300 |
| Swimming (¼ mph) | 300 |
| Walking (3¾ mph) | 300 |
| Badminton | 350 |
| Horseback riding (trotting) | 350 |
| Volleyball | 350 |
| Roller skating | 350 |
| **C. Vigorous Activity** | **over 350** |
| Table tennis | 360 |
| Ice skating (10 mph) | 400 |
| Wood chopping | 400 |
| Tennis | 420 |
| Water skiing | 480 |
| Hill climbing (100 ft. per hr.) | 490 |
| Skiing (10 mph) | 600 |
| Squash and handball | 600 |
| Cycling (13 mph) | 660 |
| Scull rowing (race) | 840 |
| Running (10 mph) | 900 |

*The standards represent a compromise between those proposed by the British Medical Association (1950), Christensen (1953) and Wells, Balke, and Van Fossan (1956). Where available, actual measured values have been used; for other values a "best guess" was made.

Data prepared by Robert E. Johnson, M.D., Ph.D., and collegues, Department of Physiology and Biophysics, University of Illinois, August, 1967 and published in a pamphlet entitled "Exercise and Weight Control."

up 900 calories, it does not have to be done all in one stretch; a half-hour, for example, uses up 450 calories.

THE PRE-GAME MEAL*

The following considerations should be factors in planning the pre-game meal:

1. Energy intake should be adequate to eliminate any feelings of weakness during the entire period of the competition. Although the pre-game meal makes only a small contribution to the body's immediate energy demands, the pre-contest food intake is essential for maintaining an adequate level of blood sugar and for avoiding the sensation of hunger.

2. The pre-game diet plan should ensure that the stomach and upper bowel are relatively empty at the time of competition.

3. Food and fluid intakes prior to and during competition should ensure an optimal state of hydration.

4. No pre-game diet should include food which will **not** upset the gastrointestinal tract.

5. In general, the pre-game meal should include food that the athlete is familiar with and is convinced will "make him win."

*Adopted from **Food for Sport** by Nathan J. Smith, M.D. (Palo Alto, California: Bull Publishing; 1976).

HOW MUCH PROTEIN IS ENOUGH?

More than any other food, protein is regarded by athletes as having desireable effects on athletic performance. The reasoning: meat is muscle; a person is what he eats; therefore, an individual can increase muscle mass and strength by eating meat. The erroneous idea that athletics increase the body's need of protein dates back to the 5th century B.C. At that time, the Greeks consumed a meat diet in the belief that it would produce stronger athletes.

Shortly after the Civil War (1866), the theory that protein is the main source of muscular energy was proven totally inaccurate. During the past 100 years, numerous studies have demonstrated that muscles burn carbohydrates and fats. Exercise simply does **not** use up protein. Therefore, no need or value exists in the consumptionof more than the amount of protein included in an average, balanced diet. If the athlete's diet includes a reasonable amount of lean meat, fish or poultry, milk and cheese, he will have **all** the protein be needs.

It is true, however, that athletes generally need substantially more calories a day during the season to maintain their weight than do their non-active peers. The need for these extra calories can best be provided by larger servings of typical foods such as bread, cereal, potatoes, rice and pasta (all carbohydrates).

## CARBOHYDRATE LOADING

Carbohydrate loading is a technique in which athletes exercise vigorously several days before athletic competition while eating a low carbohydrate diet ˙and then exercise lightly, while eating a diet very high in carbohydrates approximately 48 hours prior to competition. This technique has been shown to more than double the glycogen content of muscle and to increase the endurance of athletes. The literature is equivocal, however, about the values and potential risks associated with such technique. Additional information on carbohydrate loading is presented in Chapter 2.

## THE HAZARDS OF STARVATION

In sports such as boxing and wrestling, athletes frequently place themselves on "crash diets" combined with dehydration to make lower weight classifications. Such a practice has received widespread condemnation from various sources includin the American Medical Association. Starvation or near-starvation tends to deplete the body of certain important cell constituents which are active in the synthesis of protein. As a result, the starving athlete uses muscle tissue as a source of calories (even more than a starving non-active individual). The body fat stores are so depleted in a highly active athlete that it becomes necessary for him to draw on his body's stores of protein. Starvation can also lead to circulation impairment, ketosis, and exhaustive fatigue.

## DIETARY SUPPLEMENTS

A number of athletes believe that the ingestion of dietary supplements and/or vitamins in excess of the accepted daily standards might in some way be beneficial in meeting the additional demands imposed by exercise. There is **absolutely no evidence** to support this belief. A well balanced diet provides **all** of the calories and nutrients needed by an athlete. In fact, some vitamins are toxic and life threatening when taken in excess (vitamins A and D). In addition, there is mounting evidence against excessive consumption of vitamins E and C and nicotinic acid.

WEIGHT LOSS

Weight control can be viewed as the favorable net balance between energy in (the food an individual consumes) and energy out (the amount of energy the body uses to exist). In order to lose weight, an individual must consume less food than he utilizes as energy. Given the fact that there are approximately 3500 calories in a pound of body weight, an individual who wishes to lose two pounds a week must effect a negative weekly balance of 7000 calories. A general listing of the calorie content of typical foods is illustrated in Table 10-3.

The only way to lose weight is for the individual to either decrease the amount of food consumed or increase the amount of physical activity (or a combination of both). Regardless of the weight loss method followed, the athlete must eat a **well balanced** diet. Most of the more "popular" diets (Atkins, Stillman, etc.) are nutritionally deficient in some respect and therefore should be **avoided.** A healthy diet should include food from all four food groups every day. They are 1, milk and milk products; 2, vegetables and fruit; 3, meat, fish, poultry, eggs, and cheese; 4, bread and cereals, whole grain or enriched.

Although there is no "master diet" that will fit all athletes, there are general guidelines which can assist the individual who is interested in losing weight:

• Decrease calorie intake. If an athlete stops eating an extra 25 calories or so a day, he might stop gaining weight. And if he cuts back 100 calories a day less than his needs, he will lose 10 to 12 pounds a year.

• Learn to eat slowly and chew thoroughly.

• Limit portions of food at meals to one average serving.

• Never take second helpings.

• Omit or drastically restrict free fats—butter, margarine, mayonnaise, salad oils, cooking fats. Sufficient fat is present in lean meats, fish, poultry, eggs, and cheese to insure adequate use of the fat soluble vitamins A, D, E, and K.

• Omit or drastically restrict free sweets—jelly, jam, honey, syrups, sugar, candy, pies, pastries, and most other desserts.

• Restrict or eliminate intake of alcoholic beverages.

• Eat a good breakfast and never skip a meal.

• Never use food as a reward.

• Learn to practice moderation. If an individual decides to indulge in a high calorie food, he should eat it slowly and eat one half or less than he normally would.

## Table 10-3. Caloric values of selected foods.*

| Food | Weight or approximate measure | Calories |
|---|---|---|
| **Milk Group** | | |
| Cheese, cheddar | 1⅛ cube | 115 |
| Cheese, cottage creamed | ¼ cup | 65 |
| Cream, coffee | 1 tbsp | 30 |
| Milk, fluid, skim (buttermilk) | 1 cup | 90 |
| Milk fluid whole | 1 cup | 160 |
| **Meat Group** | | |
| Beans, dry, canned | ¾ cup | 233 |
| Beef, pot roast | 3 oz | 245 |
| Chicken | ½ breast—with bone | 155 |
| Egg | 1 medium | 80 |
| Frankfurter | 1 medium | 170 |
| Haddock | 1 fillet | 140 |
| Ham, boiled | 2 oz | 135 |
| Liver, beef | 2 oz | 130 |
| Peanut butter | 2 tbsp | 190 |
| Pork chop | 1 chop | 260 |
| Salmon, canned | ½ cup | 120 |
| Sausage, bologna | 2 slices | 173 |
| **Vegetable Group** | | |
| Beans, snap green | ½ cup | 15 |
| Broccoli | ½ cup | 20 |
| Cabbage, shredded, raw | ½ cup | 10 |
| Carrots, diced | ½ cup | 23 |
| Corn, canned | ½ cup | 85 |
| Lettuce leaves | 2 large or 4 small | 10 |
| Peas, green | ½ cup | 58 |
| Potato, white | 1 medium | 90 |
| Spinach | ½ cup | 20 |
| Squash, winter | ½ cup | 65 |
| Sweet potato | 1 medium | 155 |
| Tomato juice, canned | ½ cup (small glass) | 23 |

| Food | Weight or approximate measure | Calories |
|---|---|---|
| **Fruit Group** | | |
| Apple, raw | 1 medium | 70 |
| Apricots, dried stewed | ½ cup | 135 |
| Banana, raw | 1 medium | 100 |
| Cantaloupe | ½ melon | 60 |
| Grapefruit | ½ medium | 45 |
| Orange | 1 medium | 65 |
| Orange juice, fresh | ½ cup (small glass) | 55 |
| Peaches, canned | ½ cup with syrup | 100 |
| Pineapple juice, canned | ½ cup (small glass) | 68 |
| Prunes, dried, cooked | 5 with juice | 160 |
| Strawberries, raw | ½ cup, capped | 30 |
| **Bread-cereal Group** | | |
| Bread, white, enriched | 1 slice | 70 |
| Cornflakes, fortified | 1⅓ cup | 133 |
| Macaroni, enriched, cooked | ¾ cup | 115 |
| Oatmeal, cooked | ⅔ cup | 87 |
| Rice, cooked | ¾ cup | 140 |
| **Fats Group** | | |
| Bacon, crisp | 2 slices | 90 |
| Butter or fortified margarine | 1 tbsp | 100 |
| Oils, salad or cooking | 1 tbsp | 125 |
| **Sweets Group** | | |
| Beverages, cola type | 6 oz | 75 |
| Sugar, granulated | 1 tbsp. | 40 |

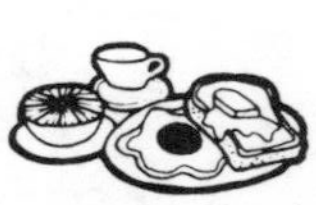

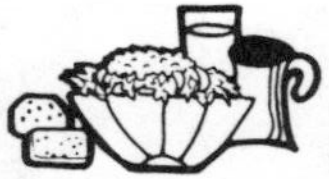

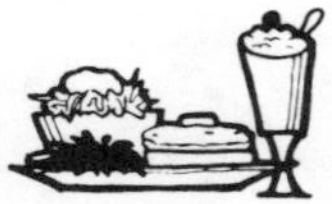

*Reprinted by permission of publisher from, **Especially for Women**, by Ellington Darden, (Leisure Press: West Point, N.Y.), 1977.

• Buy a good scale and use it. Weigh once a week and keep a written record of body weight.

• Keep a food diary. Record in detail food and drink for a week. This helps stiffen resistance to dietary temptations. It is also an important aid in that it may reveal unconscious departures.

There are a number of exercise gimmicks which purpose to aid the individual in losing weight. Ranging from inflatable clothing, vibrating machines, rubber sweatsuits, and dietary candy to weighted waist belts, these gimmicks share one commonality—**they're useless!** For example, a six foot tall, 200 pound man would have to wear a 10 pound weighted waist belt 8 hours a day for 45 days in order to shed just **one** pound.


WEIGHT GAIN

An athlete who wishes to gain functional weight (lean muscle mass), as opposed to dead weight (body fat), should engage in activities which will bulk up his musculature. The increase in weight is achieved by increasing the diameter of the individual's muscle fibers. Progressive weight training is the most effective activity for producing such a change. In this regard, training on Nautilus equipment appears to be the quickest and most efficient means for gaining weight.

# CHAPTER 11
## Injury Prevention and Treatment

Louis F. Tomasi, A.T.C.

Foot injuries
Ankle injuries
Lower leg injuries
Knee injuries
Thigh injuries
Hand injuries
Wrist injuries
Forearm injuries
Elbow injuries
Upper arm injuries
Shoulder injuries
Cervical injuries
Head injuries
Internal injuries
Head injuries

## FOOT INJURIES
### ARCH SPRAINS

**Cause**

Traumatic sprain: It is usually the result of an acute violent disruption of the plantar ligament in the longitudinal arch of the foot.

Static sprain: This problem is the result of constant stress, repetitive vigorous exercise, a change in running shoes or running surface or training techniques.

**Symptoms**

The athlete experiences pain and discomfort along the arch, inability to walk in normal fashion, and depending on the cause, a history of a traumatic incident or change in activity. There may also be swelling, point tenderness, decoloration, and some degree of arch drop.

**Treatment**

Immediate treatment is ice and elevation for the initial forty-eight hours. Thereafter, use hot whirlpools, deep heat in the form of ultrasound, arch strapping, proper fitting shoes, and/or arch support to avoid further pain and discomfort. Therapy also includes exercise to strengthen the plantar muscle. Curling a towel with the toes with weight for resistance, picking up pencils and/or marbles with the toes, and any other exercises to strengthen the plantar muscles are recommended.

## BLISTERS

Blisters on the feet are very bothersome and may pose serious medical infection if left untreated. Irregardless of the size of the blister, proper care and treatment should be taken to insure rapid recovery and freedom from infection.

### Cause

Blisters are caused by local friction between the skin and the shoe or sock. Ill fitting shoes, wrinkles in socks, or a new pair of shoes are the most common causes of blisters. Adhesive tape applied poorly to an ankle or foot may also cause "friction" blisters.

### Symptoms

The signs and symptoms of blisters are easily recognized by most people. Hot spots, pain, fluid accumulation (either blood or water) between the layers of the skin, a bubbly appearance or you may notice a blister beneath a callus.

### Treatment

The treatment of a blister may be either conservative or radical. In the conservative treatment, usually used when little or no fluid has accumulated, the closed blister is protected from further irritation by a felt or sponge rubber doughnut with the center opening large enough to surround the blister and dissipate the initial blister causing friction away from the irritated area. In the radical treatment, the blister is lanced (preferably by a physician or a trainer) and the accumulated fluid allowed to drain. As with any open wound, apply a sterile bandage and antiseptic to avoid infection.

## STRESS FRACTURES OF THE FOOT

### Cause

Fatigue or stress fractures of the foot are common among athletes involved in long-vigorous training sessions.

### Symptoms

The signs of stress fractures are chronic foot discomfort when engaging in even the slightest activity. This pain may be mistaken for arch problems. Disability and local point tenderness may also be present. Distance runners that run on hard surfaces, athletes that have purchased a new pair of shoes, or recently initiated a vigorous training program are often victims of stress fractures.

## Treatment

X-rays should be taken, although stress fractures are not always detected immediately after they occur. Stress fractures will not appear on X-ray film for three or four weeks after the acute phase. Early and proper treatment include adequate supportive measures, rest through the symptomatic phase and restricted physical activity. These procedures are a must when suspicious chronic pain of the foot is associated with vigorous training.

## TRAUMATIC FOOT FRACTURES

### Cause

This type of fracture occurs in any athletic event. It is usually caused by a crushing blow with the force delivered to a relatively small area, e.g. being stepped on by a cleat.

Foot fractures also occur in sports where leaping or jumping occurs, e.g. basketball or volleyball, where the athlete inverts the ankle. If his weight continues to turn the foot under (inversion), extreme stress is put on the fifth metatarsal, resulting in a fracture.

### Symptoms

The signs of a fracture are extreme discomfort, inability to bear weight, rapid swelling, point tenderness and a possible grinding sensation.

### Treatment

The immediate first aid is to apply ice, immobilize the fractured area (splint), elevate the leg, keep the athlete warm, and refer to the physician. Fractures are emergency situations, and they require careful handling.

## ANKLE INJURIES

### ANKLE SPRAINS

The ankle is probably the body part most often injured in physical training. Inversion sprains account for 90% of all ankle sprains. This is due to inherent instability of the skeletal structure of the ankle. Therefore, flexibility is extremely important in the execution of cutting turns, or changing lateral directions, but lends itself to ankle sprains as well.

## Cause

The ankle sprain is usually caused by a sharp inversion of the ankle joint. The ligaments on the lateral aspect are stretched, torn or ruptured depending on severity. A twisting sprain is a forced inversion of the ankle while running or walking on an uneven surface, or when landing incorrectly after a jump.

## Symptoms

The symptoms are severe pain on the outside area of the ankle gradually spreading through the entire ankle. Usually the injured athlete will be unable to bear weight in the normal manner. The degree of disability depends on the severity of ligament disruption. The athlete may also have point tenderness at the affected ligament.

## Treatment

Treatment of ankle sprains is varied. The underlying procedure that is incorporated in the treatment of ankle injuries is ice for the initial forty-eight to seventy-two hours, followed by a gradual transition to hot whirlpool, range of motion exercises, and strength development of the muscles and ligaments that surround the ankle. Rehabilitation time varies with the degree of tissue damage and can range from 5 days for mild sprains to eight to twelve weeks for more severe sprains. The following procedures are recommended in treatment of ankle sprains.

Treatment starts immediately after the injury occurs with ice, compression and elevation. The initial ice treatment is for thirty to forty-five minutes and continues at one half hour intervals. The ice or cold treatment should continue for forty-eight to seventy-two hours, with the affected limb elevated whenever possible. Hot and cold bathes or hot whirlpools should commence once the initial swelling is arrested.

Progressive resistance exercises are recommended during rehabilitation. By working in the four plans of movement, local muscle strength is increased. Walking, running, and rope skipping utilizing each leg and both legs are excellent conditioners. When the athlete cannot bear weight, bicycling on an ergometer benefits cardiovascular fitness. During the time and effort spent on reconditioning the affected limb, it is often forgotten that the body needs total conditioning as well. It is important to maintain muscular strength and cardiovascular fitness during rehabilitation to preclude new injuries upon resumptions of competition.

## EVERSION ANKLE FRACTURES

The term ankle fracture is a vague term and has many meanings.

There are many bones in the ankle joint area that may be fractured.

## Cause

The mechanics of an eversion fracture are forced eversion (outward twist) of the foot, or forced internal rotation of the lower leg on a planted foot.

## Symptoms

A forced eversion followed by pain and disability. Swelling occurs on the medial side, and subsequently spreads through the entire ankle.

## Treatment

The initial treatment of a possibly fracture is similar to the treatment used for an ankle sprain, ice, compression, elevation, immobilization and referral to a physician for X-rays.

## INVERSION ANKLE FRACTURE

## Cause

The initial cause of an inversion fracture is a forced inward twisting of the foot. The cause is similar to the mechanics involved in an inversion sprain, i.e. placing the foot upon an uneven surface and twisting the foot inward.

## Symptoms

A forced inversion of the foot, pain on the outer side of the ankle, disability, point tenderness, possible grinding sensations, and severe swelling.

## Treatment

The initial treatment of a possible fracture is ice, compression, elevation, immobilization and early referral to the hospital for X-rays. The athlete is also treated for shock that occurs in many bone fracture incidents.

## ACHILLES TENDON STRAINS

## Cause

Achilles tendon strains do occur in athletics, but their frequency of occurances is minimal. The strain is usually caused by the foot being forced back while the calf muscles are attempting to point the toe. This force may be external, as a blow to the bottom of the foot possibly caused by a flying object (to include body blocks, etc.), or internal, such as poor coordination during athletic competition.

## Symptoms

In milder strains, there is local tenderness, swelling and pain when trying to point the toe. A complete rupture results in the inability to point the toe. An acute rupture must be treated by an orthopaedic surgeon. The defect or rupture is usually felt at the musculo tendonous junction or immediately above the insertion at the calcanious or heel bone (Figure 11-1).

## Treatment

In all strains, hemorrhaging (internal bleeding) is controlled by ice compression and elevation. The athlete should continue the ice therapy for forty-eight hours. In moderate strains, crutches should be used and a heel lift inserted into the shoe to relieve the stretch on the tendon. Hot whirlpool and deep heat therapy (ultra sound) can be used when hrmorrhaging ceases.

LOWER LEG INJURIES

SHIN SPLINTS

Shin splints involve many conditions. Some of the injuries classified as shin splints that may be grouped into this category are lower leg bone stress fractures, tendonitis along the lower leg, sore, tender leg muscles and poor coordination between extensor and flexor muscles of the foot.

## Cause

The syndrome is usually initiated by excessive repeated use in an unaccustomed activity or a change in on going activity. The change may be in the running surface, shoes, style or any other changes that require adaptation. Other theories on the causes of shin splints are: inflammation of lower leg muscles; inflammation of the membrane between the bones of the lower leg; faulty standing, walking or running habits; muscle fatigue; arch disruption; improper muscle coordination between the muscle in front and behind the lower leg; abnormal stress caused by the second toe being longer than the great toe; or any combination of these factors. The theory of the larger second toe is an important aspect of shin splints. It is not necessarily a cause and affect relationship, but it is certainly a very important aspect. Athletes with a longer second toe who undertake a vigorous training program must be aware of this. It is important to insure that proper running techniques are used. The athlete should remember that it is important to point the toes in the direction of travel and push off with the big toe immediately

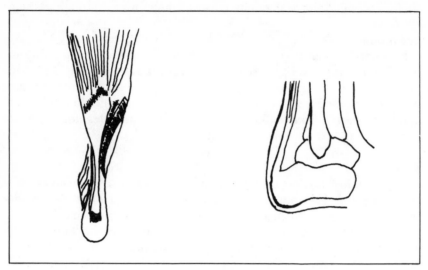

Figure 11-1. Achilles strain.

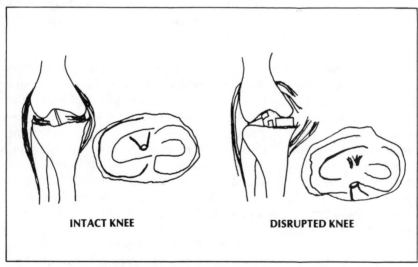

Figure 11-2. Medial ligament knee sprain.

before lifting the foot from the ground for the swing through phase of the gait.

## Symptoms

The symptoms and signs of lower leg problems are chronic pain along the front inside or outside of the lower leg, discomfort in climbing stairs, disability during training, needle point sensations along the shin, intermittant numbness in the leg, elevated shin temperature, swelling, sore to touch, shin pain when pointing the toes, and point tenderness along the surfaces of the bone. The athlete should be particularly alert for point tenderness along the outside bone of the lower leg, three to four inches above the ankle bone. This condition may be the initial signs of a stress fracture, and if present, the athlete should be referred to an orthopaedic surgeon for further evaluation.

## Treatment

The treatment of these lower leg problems vary with the various philosophies and the athlete's reactions. It is recommended that ice be applied to the painful area for the first forty-eight hours, then gradually change over to heat therapy. Heat therapy in the form of ultra sound, diathermy, or hot packs before activity, and ice, in the form of ice massage or cold whirlpools following activity are important techniques in the treatment of shin splints. Strapping the shin in an open-back basket weave fashion, and taping the arch are two techniques that alleviate the pain associated with lower leg problems.

The shoes that the athlete wears when not in activity may be a key to the successful treatment of this problem. With the shoe market flooded with "stacked" or "high-heeled" foot attire, many of the athletes are purchasing these shoes to be fashionable. These shoes put the foot in an toe pointed position which adds to the stretch already placed on the dorsiflexor muscles. The stretched position aggravates the existing condition and retards the healing process. It is recommended that the athlete avoid wearing the "stacked" heeled shoes while experiencing the symptoms of shin splints.

## KNEE INJURIES

Of all the joints in the body, the knee probably has received the most attention in the treatment of athletic injury. Strained ligaments, damaged cartilage, capsular damage, patellar dislocations, contusions, and other knee injuries have been the topic of numerous books, articles and publications. This publicity is warranted and should continue for the benefit of the athlete. Rules in football have been modifed to help reduce the number of knee injuries. The recently eliminated cut-back block by the wide receiver on the unsuspecting defensive end has shortened the careers of many football players, while clipping or hitting below the waist has been outlawed for years.

# CONTUSIONS

**Cause**

Knee contusions are usually the result of a sharp blow which damages protective soft tissue and subsequently produces swelling, disability, plus discomfort. In a simple knee contusion, the integrity of the connective tissue is not damaged. If a blow is delivered to the outside of the knee, and the sensation of pain and swelling is felt on the inside of the knee, your immediate concern should be for ligament injury. If the pain is felt on the same side that received the blow, a contusion is present.

**Symptoms**

There may be a variety of symptoms present in a knee contusion. Local swelling, tenderness at the point of contact, a black-and-blue appearance, early disappearance of the signs, and finally no disruption in the integrity of the joint are signs of a contusion.

**Treatment**

The key to full recovery from knee injury is early diagnosis and prompt, proper care. The treatment for a contusion is ice, compression and elevation until the swelling has ceased. It is imperative that the contusion be protected from further injury. A sponge rubber doughnut large enough to cover and protect the injury may be fabricated to reduce the chance of additional blows to the area when participating in athletics. The rehabilitation time is short if no further complications occur. Knee contusions, like other contusions, are self-limiting and will usually heal in a short period of time.

# MEDIAL KNEE LIGAMENT INJURY

Sprains to the knee are common in all athletics, especially contact sports. The injury producing force is delivered in a variety of ways. The injured athlete may be running, standing, lying in a pile, cutting or any number of activities that put abnormal stress on the ligaments of the knee.

**Cause**

The classic knee sprain occurs when the knee is slightly flexed, the lower leg rotated outward, the upper leg rotated inward and a strong force delivered to the outside of the knee. The severity of the injury depends on the amount of force delivered, the muscular strength, the laxity of the ligaments, and the reaction time of the athlete. Although this is the classic knee sprain, it is by no means limited to these mechanics. For instance, severe rotational shearing actions will cause cartilage to tear. Although cartilage tears are not as serious as ligament disruptions, they still demand professional care and concern.

### Symptoms
The signs and symptoms of a ligament sprain are: immediate pain, disability, instability, weakness, swelling, point tenderness at the point of disruption, laxity in the ligament, and increased mobility of the joint (wabbly knee). Because some ligaments are attached to cartilage, it is not unusual to have a cartilage tear as well as a ligament sprain (Figure 11-2).

### Treatment
The immediate treatment of a knee sprain is ice, compression and elevation. If marked instability and weakness are noted, the athlete should be examined by an orthopaedic surgeon. Depending on the severity of the sprain, the physician's action may be surgery, plaster immobilization, use of crutches, and restricted activity.

### LATERAL KNEE LIGAMENT
A sprain to the outside (lateral colateral) ligament of the knee is not uncommon in athletics. Although the incidents of lateral sprains is not as high as medial sprains, their occurance is significant.

### Cause
The injury occurs when the foot and lower leg is turned inward, the upper leg turned outward and the injury-producing force delivered to the inside of the knee.

### Symptoms
The outside part of the knee is the location of pain, swelling, weakness, instability, and laxity. Point tenderness may also be present at the location of the disruption. The severity of the injury varies from a stretching of fibers to a complete rupture of the ligament.

### Treatment
Immediate treatment is identical to the medial sprain, ice, compres-

sion, elevation, and orthopaedic surgeon consultation in the more severe cases.

## MEDIAL CARTILAGE INJURY

### Cause

Knee cartilage injuries are associated with torsion or twisting of the upper and lower leg in opposite direction. A forced internal rotation of the thigh bone upon a stationary lower leg may result in a knee cartilage tear. This type of tear is commonly referred to as a "bucket handle" tear.

### Symptoms

In cartilage tears, there is swelling, functional pain, an audible clicking or snapping sensation in the knee, insecurity (a "give-way" feeling), disability, local pain at the inside joint line, limited range of motion, and pain elicited on forced extension.

### Treatment

The immediate treatment of a cartilage sprain is ice, compression and elevation. When there is uncertainty concerning the extent of the injury, the athlete should consult a physician or an orthopaedic surgeon.

## LATERAL KNEE CARTILAGE INJURY

### Cause

Forced bending of the knee with the lower leg externally rotated, as in squatting or duck waddle-type exercise, inflicts abnormal stress on the lateral cartilage and may result in a tear. When the foot is firmly planted and the thigh is rotated outward upon the lower leg, a cartilage tear is also highly probable.

### Symptoms

The symptoms are similar to those described previously in the medial cartilage sprain section.

### Treatment

The immediate care for a suspected cartilage tear is ice, compression, elevation and early referral to a physician.

## PATELLAR (KNEE CAP) DISRUPTIONS

### Cause

Patellar dislocations or partial dislocations occur in all sports. The cause of a patellar disruption is a violent force delivered against the inside edge of the patella when the thigh is rotated on a planted foot. A violent contraction of the thigh muscle may also cause a patella to dislocate. Picture the patella as a paper clip attached at a mid-point of a rubberband that is attached at the hip and just-below the knee. The angle formed by the "rubberband" between the thigh and lower leg approximates a straight line in a man, while the woman's forms an angle less than 180°. As the woman's thigh muscle is suddenly contracted (the rubberband stretched), the force of the contraction dislocates the patella in a lateral direction, much like the paper clip would move in that direction. It is hypothesized that this phenomenon accounts for the higher rate of patella dislocations in the female population.

### Symptoms

There is usually severe pain and point tenderness along the inside border of the knee cap. There may also be an indentation, swelling, muscle spasm, and disability. In many incidents, the patella spontaneously relocates itself, but there will still be the aforementioned symptoms.

### Treatment

In many dislocations, the patella reduces itself. In any case, the leg should be immobilized, packed in ice, and referred to a physician. Immobilization is recommended for four weeks and in some cases even longer. Physical therapy is required to rebuild the strength in the affected leg. Rehabilitation consists of straight leg raises in all four directions, with gradual progression to resistive and range of motion exercise, i.e. isokinetic or isotonic exercise.

### REHABILITATION FOR THE KNEE

A rehabilitation program starts with straight leg lifts, increased range of motion exercises, progressive, resistive or isokinetic exercises, slow straight running, slow figure 8 running, agility drills, and, with progress, a progressively intensified program. Rehabilitation programs are found in many athletic trainer's publications.

## THIG H INJURIES

## CONTUSIONS

### Cause

The quadricep muscle group (thigh muscles) is particularly prone to contusions in many sports. Thigh contusions are usually a result of a direct force applied locally to the thigh muscle. The force is delivered by a jarring tackle when contact is made with the shoulder pads, helmet, knee, elbow, or any other instrument that applies force to compress the muscle tissue against the femur. (This type injury is commonly called a Charlie Horse).

## Symptoms

The symptoms and signs are point tenderness, limited range of motion, presence of a hematoma caused by internal bleeding, pain, and difficulty in movement, and possibly a downward movement of the hematoma.

## Treatment

Treatment of a contusion must be immediate. The "shaking off" of a thigh contusion (continue to play) increases internal bleeding and delays the healing process. With the injured muscle stretched, ice is applied directly to the injury site for forty-five minutes. A compression wrap using a foam rubber pad slightly larger than the injured area may also be utilized to reduce the size of the hematoma. Elevation of the injured leg retards local swelling. The cold compression wrap must be continuously applied with a thirty minute on and thirty minute off rotation for the remainder of the day. Nightly elevation, continuous ice applications, and the use of crutches for four to seven days reduces the possibility of reoccuring internal bleeding.

Heat therapy should be used only after the hematoma starts to reduce. Whirlpool treatment should proceed a running or weight training program. Do not hesitate to regress to ice and compression at the first incidence of re-swelling. Ice will retard the swelling, and the rehabilitation process may proceed.

## MYOSITIS OSSIFICANS (CALCIUM DEPOSITS)

### Cause

Myositis ossificans or calcium deposits develop with repeated blows or irritation to a thigh contusion. With repeated blows or too early initiated activity after injury, calcification of the hematoma may develop leaving an ossified mass (calcium deposit) to complicate and hinder the healing process.

**Symptoms**
The initial signs are prolonged pain and disability, an immobile-firm mass, limited range of motion, and deep muscular pain. The mass usually shows up as a shadow on X-ray films within three to four weeks.

**Treatment**
Proper therapy and avoiding activity too early after injury are the best procedures to reduce the possibility of calcium deposits in the thigh area. When the symptoms are recognized, it is important to consult a physician.


## HAND INJURIES

### FRACTURES

**Symptoms**
The initial signs are disability, pain, point tenderness, or a grinding sensation.

**Treatment**
When a finger fracture is suspected, the finger should be splinted in the partially flexed position. This is accomplished by placing a splint on the finger, and immobilizing the joint above and below the fracture. Early referral to an orthopaedic surgeon is recommended.


### MALLET FINGER

**Cause**
"Mallet finger" fractures occur commonly in sports such as baseball, football, rugby or basketball. The fracture usually occurs when a player attempts to catch the ball, and it strikes the tip of the finger forcing it to flex while the tendons are attempting to extend the finger.

**Symptoms**
The signs of a mallet finger are first joint displacement, point tenderness and swelling. The athlete is unable to fully extend the tip of the injured finger because of the detached tendon.

**Treatment**
When a mallet finger is recognized, it should be splinted in the hyperextended position and referred to a physician. Recovery time for this injury is usually four to six weeks.

## FINGER AND THUMB SPRAIN

**Cause**

The joints of the fingers and thumbs are particularly prone to sprains. The injury producing force usually causes hyperextension. Thumb and finger sprains occur most often in activities that involve catching a ball, football, volleyball, basketball or baseball.

**Symptoms**

The signs of a thumb sprain are pain in the joint, swelling, limited range of motion, and inability to touch the little finger with the thumb. In a chronic occurance, there is a recurrent weakness of the ligaments and the muscles of the thumb.

**Treatment**

Immediate application of ice compression, elevation, follow-up ice treatments, gradual transition to heat and adequate strapping to avoid further injury, is recommended in the treatment of this injury.

## FINGER AND THUMB DISLOCATIONS

**Cause**

Dislocations are usually the result of a force delivered to the end of the digit causing it to dislocate. The force usually causes a disruption of the second joint resulting in a dislocation.

**Symptoms**

The signs of a dislocation are pain, limited range of motion, obvious deformity, swelling, and tenderness.

**Treatment**

Reduction is accomplished by exerting a force along the bone ends, pushing the heads of the bone away from the joint. The joint will reduce with less damage to the connective tissue when the digit is reduced. Pack it in ice and seek medical attention for X-ray examination.

## THUMB FRACTURES

**Cause**

Thumb fractures occur frequently in athletics. The fracturing force is usually a crushing one that fractures the bone along the shaft of the bone. The fracture may be caused by a crashing shoulder pad, helmet, a twisting action, or a hyperextension suffered in a fall when an outstretched thumb is bent the wrong way.

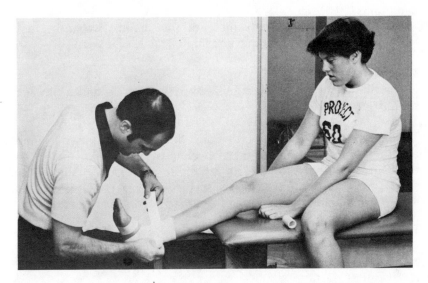

Proper taping can reduce the incidence of several kinds of injuries.

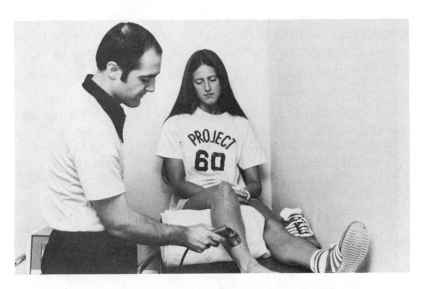

Ultra-sound is one of the best methods of treating "shin splints."

## Symptoms
Pain associated with movement of the thumb, weakness, point tenderness, disability, swelling, and limited range of motion.

## Treatment
The thumb should be immobilized, packed in ice and a physician should be consulted.

Note: The thumb is an important digit of the hand. It is used in almost all grips. Improper or inadequate healing of a fractured thumb may result in a disability for life. If a fracture, dislocation, subluxation, sprain, or strain to the thumb is suspected, proper conservative treatment is usually rewarded by significant and successful retention of the normal thumb movement and use.

## LONG HAND BONE FRACTURES

### Cause
Metacarpal (hand bone) fractures are usually caused by a direct blow either to the end of the bone, the shaft, or the neck.

### Symptoms
The fracture is recognized by point tenderness, local pain, swelling, and referred pain at the fracture site when tapping pressure is applied along the long axis of the metacarpal. Additional signs of a fracture are a shortening of the metacarpal, a grinding sensation, and an obvious deformity in the hand.

### Treatment
Proper treatment of a suspected long bone fracture of the hand is of great importance. It must be treated carefully to avoid soft tissue, neurological or blood vessel damage. The fracture should be splinted and wrapped to immobilize the joint above and below the fracture sites. The athlete should see an orthopaedic surgeon for proper alignment and plaster immobilization as soon as possible after the injury.

Note: A fracture that occurs frequently in boxing affects the fourth and/or fifth metacarpal. The fracture is caused by the improper execution of a punch resulting in the impact affecting the heads of 4th and/or 5th metacarpals. The fractured metacarpal will sometimes displace resulting in a disformity of the palm of the hand. The impact may also be transmitted down the shaft causing it to fracture.

## WRIST INJURIES
## SPRAINS AND FRACTURES

**Cause**

Hyperextension and hyperflexion sprains, strains and fractures are probably the most common athletic injuries to the wrist. These injuries usually occur by falling on the outstretched hand, or excessive force applied to the palm of the hand.

**Symptoms**

In a hyperextension sprain, the hand is usually forced past normal extension resulting in pain, swelling and possible numbness of the wrist. When the fall is very severe, the carpal bones may transfer the force to the navicular bone in the wrist resulting in a fracture to its narrowest point. The lunat bone in the mid-wrist may also dislocate resulting in pain, discomfort, pressure in the carpal tunnel and numbness in the finger. There may also be a palpatable depression on the posterior side of the wrist and a bulge on the anterior side of the wrist.

**Treatment**

Many wrist fractures are frequently diagnosed as bad sprains. It is recommended that X-rays be taken of all severe wrist injuries. Even if X-rays are negative, the possibility of navicular fracture still exists if the symptoms persist. Incomplete healing caused by a poor blood supply will delay bone healing for as long as one year. Cases of plaster immobilization for as long as one year do occur. Sprained wrists that fail to heal within 6 to 8 weeks should be suspicious and once again referred for X-ray.

## FOREARM INJURIES
## FOREARM SPLINTS

**Cause**

Forearm splints are like shin splints and are caused by minute disruptions in the membrane between the forearm bones (ulna and radius) brought about by an occluded blood supply. The problem is likely to occur in gymnastics, particularly among those gymnasts that execute arm supportive stunts. It is also hypothesized that forearm splints are minute muscle tears caused by continuous stress placed on the forearm muscles.

**Symptoms**

The signs of forearm splints are dull aching pains in the forearm, weakness, and chronic pain.

**Treatment**
If these symptoms appear early in the season, moist heat, deep heat in the form of ultra sound, and rest are all the proper forms of therapy. If the symptoms appear late in the season, strapping with tape and therapy may help the athlete survive the final events.

## CONTUSIONS

**Cause**
Contusions of the forearm frequently occur in rugby and football players. In football, the contusion is usually the result of the player throwing his forearm into the pads or face mask of an opponent.

**Symptoms**
The forearm contusion will immediately swell, restrict active motion, be stiff, and usually a hematoma will develop.

**Treatment**
Ice, compression, elevation and restrictive motion retards the swelling. Padding and strapping precludes re-injury to the athlete's arm during recovery. If a contusion is treated incorrectly, and the athlete resumes competition too soon, calcification of the damaged tissue mass may result, rendering the athlete inactive until the mass reabsorbs.

## FRACTURES

**Cause**
A radial or ulna fracture occurs when a direct force is delivered to the forearm. The force may be the blow from a stick, or an attempted tackle where the arm is caught between the moving legs of a running back. Falling on an outstretched arm may also fracture one or both of the forearm bones. In this type of fracture, forearm bones may be jammed resulting in a telescopic fracture of the radius. Although rare, this is one of the many injuries that may occur when athletes are unaccustomed to falling or fall incorrectly. The athlete reaches out the arm to cushion his impact to the ground or mat, and the force is dissipated at the end of the forearm bone causing injury.

**Symptoms**
A fracture in the forearm may occur to either or both of the forearm bones (radius or ulna). The signs and symptoms are the same as other long bone fractures, pain, swelling, possible deformity, and disability. Finger numbness, limited rotational action of the lower arm, and

210

temporary loss of function of the hand are additional signs of this type injury.

## ELBOW INJURIES
### HYPEREXTENSION

**Cause**

Hyperextention injuries to the elbow occur most frequently in boxing and wrestling. The mechanics of the injury are similar in both sports, but the causes are different. In boxing the most frequent cause is a thrown punch that misses. The punch is thrown with the force to make contact with the opponent near complete extension. When the opponent eludes the punch, hyperextension of the elbow results. Ligament tears are also common in such injuries.

The wrestling injury is caused by falling on an outstretched arm either with the athlete's weight or the weight of both wrestlers. Forced hyperextension may also be caused by a missed move, or counter-move, illegal hold, etc.

**Symptoms**

The signs and symptoms of an elbow hyperextension are pain on the inside of the elbow, swelling, disability, point tenderness along the inside colateral ligaments plus the inability and little desire to fully extend the elbow.

**Treatment**

Immediate first aid is the application of ice and elevation for forty-eight hours, then a gradual transition to heat therapy. When the athlete continues athletic participation, strapping the arm to prevent hyperextension is recommended to avoid further injury to the elbow.

### ELBOW BURSITIS

**Cause**

Elbow or Olecranon bursitis is caused by a direct blow to the back of the elbow. The bursa's location immediately beneath the skin makes it susceptible to acute or chronic contusions. The blow may be caused by a fall onto that area, or being struck with an implement.

**Symptoms**

Pain, swelling, and a rise in local skin temperature are the signs of bursitis disruption.

## Treatment

Immediate treatment for elbow bursitis involves ice, compression, elevation and cessation of activity.

## DISLOCATIONS

### Cause

The usual cause of a dislocated elbow is falling on an outstretched hand with the arm extended. The hand, wrist, and forearm remains stationary, but the upper arm bone (humerus) continues in the downward direction departing the notch it usually fits into and comes to rest on the ulna. (Figure 11-3).

### Symptoms

When an elbow is dislocated there is severe swelling, pain, disability and the elbow fixed in moderate flexion or extension. In the posterior dislocation, more common, the point of the elbow is prominent. In an anterior dislocation, the elbow point is lost. The appearance of the elbow indicates it is obviously malaligned. Elbow dislocations involve extensive ligament damage, plus it is accompanied by hemorrhaging, possible circulatory and/or neurological disruptions.

### Treatment

Emergency treatment for a dislocated elbow is to apply ice, compression and elevation. Absence of a radial pulse indicates occluded or impaired blood supply and transportation to a medical facility must be accelerated. The athlete should also be tested for sensory and motor functions of the hand to determine if any neurological damage has occured, e.g. a hand drop. Setting a dislocated elbow is accomplished by a physician, and the time lapse between dislocation and setting should by minimal to avoid extensive tissue damage. Immobilization and sling suspension is usually prescribed for approximately three weeks. Gradual range of motion, forearm flexion exercises and hydrotherapy are used for rehabilitation. A too strenuous or too early rehabilitation program may result in a calcium build-up in the elbow.

## UPPER ARM INJURIES
### (HUMERAL) FRACTURES

### Cause

The causes of an upper arm or humeral fracture is similar to the elbow dislocation; falling on the outstretched arm, a direct violent force, or a fall onto the upper arm.

## Symptoms

An upper arm fracture near the elbow may be mistaken for an elbow dislocation; therefore, the complications associated with a fractured humerus are similar to a dislocated elbow. An upper arm fracture will cause a hand-wrist drop and a blueish color in the hand.

## Treatment

The immediate treatment is ice, compression and elevation with expediant transportation to medical authorities.

The elbow is an important joint in the body and, unfortunately, often injured. If these injuries are handled professionally, judiously, and prudently, then rehabilitation should go smoothly, and the possibility of complications will be minimized.

## SHOULDER INJURIES

Shoulder injuries occur frequently in many sports. Falling on an outstretched arm, forced hyperextension, direct lateral force, or falling on the point of the shoulder are some of the factors that contribute to injured shoulders. The injuries that occur most frequently are acromiuclavicular (AC) sprains, dislocated gleno-humeral joint, subluxating shoulder and rotator cuff tears.

## SHOULDER A-C SPRAINS

### Cause

The A-C separation injury occurs in one of two ways: the athlete falls on the point of the shoulder driving the acromeon process of the scapula down; or, falling on an outstretched arm with the arm close to a slightly in front of the body.

### Symptoms

Depending on the severity, the signs and symptoms are shoulder pain, disability, point tenderness, elevated clavical or depressed scapula, ligamentous laxity, and relief with sling suspension. In an A-C sprain, the coracoclavicular (CC) ligament may also be involved which will account for the elevated clavicle (Figure 11-4).

### Treatment

Immediate care for the AC sprain is ice, sling and swatch, and early referral to an orthopaedic surgeon in moderate to severe cases.

Rehabilitation of an AC separation is dependent on the severity of the injury. Ice and pressure are used for forty-eight to seventy-two hours

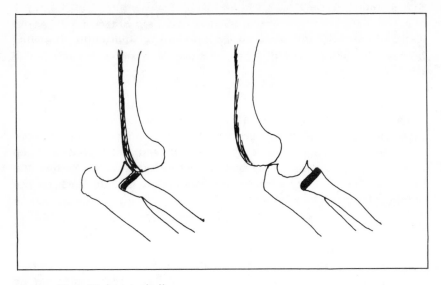

Figure 11-3. Dislocated elbow.

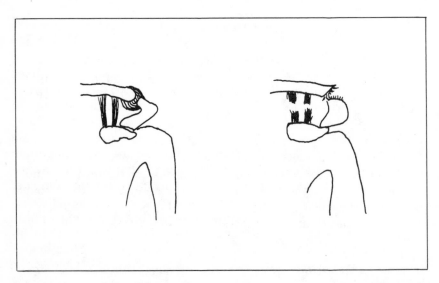

Figure 11-4. A-C shoulder sprain.

with a gradual transition to heat and deep heat therapy, if no surgery is required. Range of motion exercises may begin as soon as the sub-acute phase has passed. Similar to all the previous rehabilitation programs, constant orthopaedic surgeon-therapist-trainer rapport is needed.

## DISLOCATIONS

### Cause
Shoulder dislocations are common in sports that involve the shoulder complex. Falling on the outstretched arm or a force applied to an abducted and/or external rotated arm is severe enough to tear the capsular ligaments resulting in the relocation of the head of the humerus. Arm tackling, the backstroke in swimming, the switch in wrestling, or reaching up and behind when rebounding in basketball are prime examples of the mechanics of injury.

### Symptoms
The signs of a shoulder dislocation are pain and disability; the symptoms of a shoulder dislocation are the arm fixed in abduction and external rotation, loss of the round shoulder appearance, prominent acromion, and the inability to touch the opposite shoulder with the affected arm's hand.

### Treatment
When a dislocation occurs, reduction by the orthopaedic surgeon is required and should be accomplished as quickly as possible. In many instances, the surgeon is not immediately available; therefore, rapid transportation to the physician is necessary. It is wise to telephone ahead to the hospital to inform the emergency room of the situation. Complications that may arise with a dislocated shoulder are loss of blood flow, nerve severance, or a fractured humerus or scapula.

Rehabilitation may begin when range of motion exercises are pain free. The internal rotators of the humerus are the most important muscles during rehabilitative strength training. That is not to say the other motions are not important. Horizontal and anterior shoulder flexion, abduction, plus the other motions, must also be strengthened. Physical therapy includes hydroccolator packs, diathermy and/or ultra sound. It is safe for the athlete to resume normal activity when his strength is back to normal (about three to five weeks). Strapping or taping is recommended in severe or chronic cases of shoulder dis-locations.

## ROTATOR CUFF TEARS

**Cause**

A rotator cuff strain occurs to the muscle on the top and back of the shoulder. They are usually caused by falling on the outstretched arm or forced abduction of the arm.

**Symptoms**

The stretching of muscle fibers, the amount of pain, disability, weakness, grinding noise, and shoulder motion disruption are dependent on the traumatic force and the athlete's physical strength at the time of the incident. Because it is a muscular disruption, active resistance and passive stretching will produce pain.

**Treatment**

Ice, temporary sling suspension, and a gradual transition to the heat modalities is the recommended treatment. A conservative approach to rotator cuff tears prevents excessive scar adhesions, reoccurance, and a smoother road to recovery.

## CERVICAL INJURIES

Cervical injuries have received a great deal of attention in the past few years. The increasing number of injuries in this area is of concern to physicians, trainers, physical educators, parents and athletes. In recent years, legal action has even been taken against coaches for teaching "lead with the head" tackling techniques.

**Cause**

The mechanics of a cervical injury are numerous. Hyperextension, hyperflexion, forced lateral flexion and/or rotation, spearing or hitting with the crown of the head, are but a few of the forces that cause cervical injury. The athlete should always be aware of neck injuries in the contact or collision sports. Prevention of cervical injuries may be accomplished by building strong neck muscles, readiness of the athlete to absorb a cervical stress, and good officiating that prohibits spearing or head first contact in football.

The most serious injury that occurs to the neck is a cervical vertebral fracture. The mechanics of the injury are severe hyperextension, flexion and/or rotational forces. When the neck is hyperextended, the spinal processes are forced together possibly resulting in a compression fracture of the processes.

## Symptoms

The signs and symptoms of cervical disruption are pain, muscle spasm, numbness, neck stiffness, point tenderness, evidence of a damaged spinal cord, affected reflexes, tingling in extremities, and possible paralysis below the site of the injury. Forced hyperextension and hyperflexion are two types of motion that cause cervical injuries.

## Treatment

When cervical injury is suspected, do not move the athlete excessively. If at all possible, wait for professional attention, excessive movement or unprofessional administration of first aid may result in further injury. An orthopaedic surgeon should be seen as soon as possible.

## NECK STINGERS

### Cause

The nerve stretch syndrome is an injury that is prevalent in wrestling, rugby, football, hockey and other contact sports. The mechanics of the injury are hypermobility and/or torsion in the neck. Another common occurance is the depressing of the shoulder coupled with the lateral flexion of the neck in the opposite direction.

### Symptoms

The initial signs of an injury are firey, burning or needle point sensations through the shoulder and arm, and temporary paralysis extending to the fourth and fifth fingers. The symptoms are unilateral muscle spasm, limited range of motion, loss of strength in making a fist, pain, and eventually atrophy (shrinking) in the trapezius muscles. It is important in cervical nerve injuries to check for atrophy. This loss of muscular strength leaves the athlete susceptible to more serious neck injuries; therefore, 100% recuperation is recommended before the athlete returns to full competition.

### Treatment

On the first occurance of a nerve stretch injury, it is important that the athlete obtain the proper medical attention. Once the physician has diagnosed the problem therapy is initiated. Moist heat, deep heat therapy, cervical traction, bed rest, range of motion exercises, ice massage, and other treatments are used in less serious cervical nerve injuries.

## HEAD INJURIES

### Cause

Head injuries present special problems in athletics. A blow to the head is the usual cause of a head injury. Because of the close proximity of the brain, head injuries are **serious injuries** and must be regarded as potentially life threatening.

### Symptoms and Treatment

The first step in the treatment of head injuries is to establish an airway to maintain proper ventilation. Make sure the tongue or dental fixtures are free of the airway. Prevent excessive head movement.

The presence of fluid dripping from the nose or ear are symptoms of serious head injuries. Unilateral pupil dilation, lack of reaction to light, non-coordinated eye movement, impaired vision, decreasing pulse rate, increasing blood pressure, and nausea are additional symptoms of a serious head injury.

Although mild concussions seldom present any side effects, a moderate concussion poses a more serious medical problem. In a moderate concussion, the victim is usually temporarily unconscious, has a headache, impaired vision or balance, tinnitus (ringing in ears), possible personality changes, and impaired neurological signs. The moderate concussion may have many complications, and for this reason when unconsciousness occurs, a medical examination and hospitalization is strongly recommended.

A severe concussion represents a medical emergency. Extended unconsciousness and severe indications of any of the aforementioned symptoms indicate that the athlete needs medical assistance immediately.

When an athlete sustains a moderate or severe concussion, the individual should be removed from contact sports for at least three weeks or longer depending on the severity of the injury. In moderate cases, the athlete may begin participating in sports again within two to three weeks by light running. If the recovery progresses well, the intensity and duration of athletic participation may be increased. If an athlete sustains three significant concussions, he is susceptible, and future participation in contact sports is questionable.

Head injuries are a significant problem in athletics. Unfortunately, such injuries occur all to frequently. Proper coaching techniques, use of protective equipment, and prudent participation in athletics go a long way in guarding against these unfortunate injuries.

INTERNAL INJURIES

## SPLEEN INJURIES

Internal injuries to a vital organ of the body may be serious and tragic in nature. The injury that is of utmost concern is a spleenic injury.

**Cause**

Spleenic injuries are caused by a blow to the left thoracic area. Contact sports and sports played with sticks (lacrosse, hockey) produce the greatest amount of these injuries in athletics. Athletes with suspected or confirmed infectious mononucleosis are particularly susceptible to injury because while they have this disease their spleen is enlarged and very fragile. A blow delivered to the area of the spleen may rupture it.

**Symptoms**

Pain in the spleenic area, nausea, weakness, abdominal pain, white skin color, rigid or tight abdominal muscles, slowing heart rate, falling blood pressure, unconsciousness, shock and possibly cardiac arrest are all symptoms of spleenic injury.

**Treatment**

This is a medical emergency, and the actions must be undertaken immediately. If no ambulance is around, the athlete should be made comfortable, treated for shock, and transported to the hospital as soon as possible. To forewarn the hospital of the incident, someone should telephone ahead to the emergency room. This action will save precious minutes and possibly save the life of the injured athlete.

HEAT INJURIES

**Cause and Temperature Regulation**

Football is the one sport that seems to incur the majority of heat injuries. The athletes return to the campus in mid-August to participate in preseason football. The prime candidate is an interior lineman who is overweight, in poor physical condition, and spent the entire summer working in an air conditioned environment. When this athlete is exposed to the hot-humid days of late summer, with temperatures of greater than 90°F and relative humidity of greater than 40%, a heat injury will most likely occur. Ironically, heat injuries also occur at relatively low temperatures, such as 60°F, when the relative humidity is high (90% to 100%).

When an athlete initiates physical activity, various metabolic processes are increased. This increase in activity results in an increase in the body core temperature. When the core temperature increases, heat transfers from the vital organs to the blood. The blood transports the core heat to the skin blood vessels. The skin, cooled by evaporation of perspiration, facilitates heat transfer because of the increased thermal gradient between the skin and blood. The cooled blood returns to the core to further relieve the body of heat.

If the relative humidity and temperature is high, and the air is saturated and unable to accept additional moisture, problems can and often do arise. When the sweat is not evaporated the skin surface is not cooled and blood, carrying core heat to the skin surface, is not cooled. Consequently, heat is returned to the body core and the thermal regulatory systems is hindered. If the body cannot dissipate heat because of restrictive clothing, the problems are compounded. The internal body temperature continues to rise with no outlet and severe heat injury can easily occur.

**Symptoms**

The symptoms and signs of heat injury are the keys to early recognition and emergency care. These signs are not absolute. Several combinations of symptoms may be exhibited. Heat casualties may progress from one level of severity to another in a very short period of time. The course of heat injury does not always follow a set pattern. Heat injury is a life-death situation and must be treated appropriately. Excessive water loss and heat cramps frequently proceed the heat problem. The symptoms and signs of heat illness are:

Heat Exhaustion

Symptoms — Fatigue, listlessness, faintness, heart palpitations, nausea, vomiting, headache, dizziness, vertigo, shortness of breath, obstructed vision, hyperventilation, and cramps;

Signs — shock, profuse sweating, weak and rapid pulse, low blood presure, ashen in color, wet skin;

Heat Stroke

Symptoms — sensation of extreme heat, mental confusion, headache, vertigo, intolerance to light, collapse:

Signs — cessation of sweating, hot-dry skin, high fever, low blood pressure, rapid and weak pulse, slow tendon response, dilation of pupils, deliria, comatose, and labored breathing.

Emergency Care and Treatment

The immediate first aid of a heat problem may be the most important step in the recovery.

At the first sign do not discuss what should be done, DO IT.

1. Remove clothing without delay.

2. Cool body either with hose, shower, ice, anything.

3. Give electrolyte fluids in sips, as the athlete requests.

4. Get to proper medical attention rapidly and inform the medical authorities of your suspicions.

5. Continue to cool the athlete enroute to the hospital, using ice applied to the chest, neck, shoulder, face and torso area.

6. Lower body temperature then cover with blanket to avoid chills.

7. Continue to administer fluids.

Prevention

The adage "an ounce of prevention is worth a pound of care" is very important when referring to heat illnesses. This potential danger should be a major concern to athletes when activity occurs on hot-humid days.

It is also an excellent idea for athletes to use a weight chart to monitor their weight. If an athlete loses 5% to 10% of his body weight during practice, and he has not replenished that weight by the next practice session, then he is a prime candidate for heat injury. The weight lost is from fluids, which should be replaced before the individual participates again.

# CHAPTER 12
## Muscle Tonus Exercises

Susan L. Peterson
Director of Self-Defense for Women

Abdominals
Trunk
Hips

Although athletes may generally be in good physical condition, some muscle areas of their bodies may be slack, lacking firmness and tonus. Muscle tonus exercises are designed to firm, shape and contour muscles. Although these exercises will not result in spot reducing or massive losses in body weight, muscle tonus exercises **will improve** girth measurements which in turn will improve the fit of clothing. The exercises within this chapter emphasize those body areas in which men and women typically experience tonus loss: abdominals; trunk; and the hips (buttocks and upper legs).

Muscle tonus exercises should be performed slowly and smoothly. A general rule in performance would be 2 counts (count 1001, 1002,) for movement upward and 4 counts (count 1001, 1002, 1003, 1004) for movement downward. The minimum number of repetitions should be 6 to 8 and the maximum 20 to 25. Ideally, the exercises are performed daily. At the minimum, the number of work-outs should be no less than 3 times a week.

Warm-up exercises which increase circulation and raise muscle temperature should be performed at the beginning of any exercise program. Warm-ups prepare the body for strenuous muscular activity and help to prevent injuries. These warm-ups should include slow stretching for those muscle groups which will subsequently be discussed in this chapter.

With regular exercise, improvements should be noticed within 4-6 weeks. Improvements will occur, however, only if the exercises are performed correctly and regularly. Due to different individual characteristics, the same muscle tonus exercises may effect body measurements in a diversified manner among individuals. Muscle tonus improvement will depend solely upon the individual's desire and expended effort to exercise correctly.

ABDOMINALS (Stomach)

### CURL-UPS

**Starting Position:** Back lying, knees bent, feet flat on the floor, and

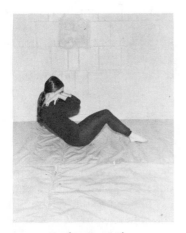

**Curl-ups:** action

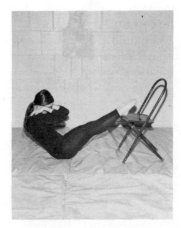

**Curl-ups**: variation # 1 — action

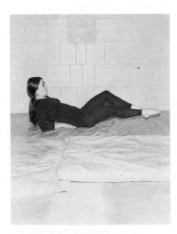

**Horizontal Bicycle Sequence:** action (center position)

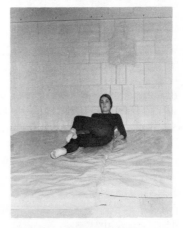

**Horizontal Bicycle Sequence:** action (side position)

fingers interlaced behind the head or resting on the shoulders.

**Action:** Tuck chin to chest and slowly curl up raising head, shoulders, and upper back off floor—do not come to a full situp position—pause and slowly uncurl back but do not touch the floor. Immediately repeat the curl-up.

Variation I: S.P.—rest extended legs on the edge of a chair, bed, or table. Do curl-up.

Variation II: Action—curl-up and hold that position for 15-30 seconds, uncurl—pause—and repeat.

## HORIZONTAL BICYCLE SEQUENCE

**Starting Position:** Back lying with upper body supported back on forearms. Lower back stays in contact with the floor—do not arch the back?

**Action:** Raise legs up off floor 6-10". Slightly bend one knee as the other leg moves forward and slightly off floor; alternate legs slowly and repeat in a bicycle pedaling fashion. Pedal center 6 counts. Immediately roll onto right hip (head and shoulders facing forward) and pedal right 6 counts; return center and pedal 6 counts; roll left and pedal 6 counts; return center pedaling 6 counts and rest. Repeat sequence C, R, C, L, C, etc.

## LOW DOUBLE LEG RAISE

**Starting Position:** Back lying with upper body supported back on forearms. Toes are extended. Do not arch the lower back!

**Action:** Slowly raise both legs up off floor only 12"-15", pause and slowly lower but not all the way to the floor, pause and repeat raise.

Note: The legs are not raised to a full vertical position.

TRUNK (Waist)

## TRUNK ROTATING SITUPS

**Starting Position:** Bent knee sitting, feet flat on floor, and fingers interlaced behind head or resting on the shoulders.

**Action:** Rotate the trunk as far right as possible and slowly uncurl backwards but do not rest on the floor; pause and remaining in rotation, slowly curl upward. Immediately repeat rotation to the left and repeat curl.

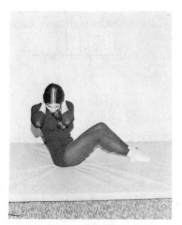

**Trunk Rotating Situps:**
action

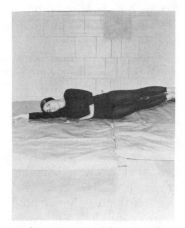

**Side Lying Dougle Leg Lift:**
action

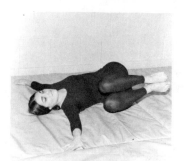

**Hip Roll Leg Extension:**
action #1

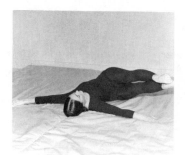

**Hip Roll Leg Extension:**
action #2

## SIDE LYING DOUBLE LEG LIFT

**Starting Position:** Side lying, legs extended one on top of the other with feet parallel to floor and ankles flexed up toward lower leg.

**Action:** Slowly raise both legs off floor and hold 6 counts. Slowly lower legs but do not rest on floor. Immediately repeat up and down. Repeat on other side of body.

Note: Keep the body in a straight position, not rolling forward onto stomach or backward onto buttocks.

## HIP ROLL LEG EXTENSION

**Starting Position:** Back lying, legs extended and arms held out to sides at shoulder level.

**Action:** Slowly bend knees up to chest, then roll right with knees pointed toward right elbow and lower knees 1-2" from floor. Immediately extend legs diagonally right and hold just off floor for 6 counts. Bend knees and return center. Roll left, extend and hold 6 counts; return center, R, C, L, etc.

Note: Keep head, shoulders, and upper back on floor as much as possible. Also do not arch the back while legs are extended and held!

HIPS (Buttocks and Upper Legs)
## REVERSE HAND KNEE LEG LIFT

**Starting Position:** Reverse hand-knee position (hands and feet flat on floor) with hips held up high level with shoulders.

**Action:** Extend right leg out up off floor with toes pointed and raise to hip level, pause and slowly lower but not all the way to the floor. Immediately repeat lift in succession. Repeat with left leg.

## HAND KNEE LEG LIFT

**Starting Position:** Hand knee stand on all fours.

**Action:** Extend right leg backwards slightly off floor with toes pointed and slowly lift to hip level, then slowly lower but do not touch the floor. Repeat in succession. Repeat with left leg.

## HAND-KNEE EXTENDED LEG LIFT

**Starting Position:** Hand knee stand on all fours.

**Action:** Slowly extend right leg backward and upward toward ceiling so weight moves forward over hands and left knee. Quickly press backward

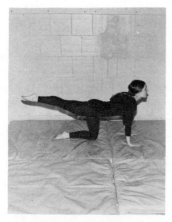

**Hand Knee Leg Lift:** action

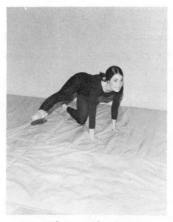

**Lateral Leg Lift:** action

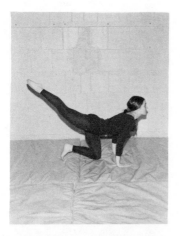

**Hand Knee Extended Leg
Lift:** starting position

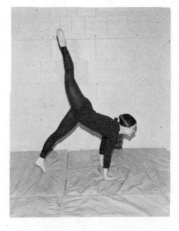

**Hand Knee Extended Leg
Lift:** action

with left foot, lifting and extending left knee and leg to raise the body while holding right leg high. Slowly return to starting position and repeat.

## LATERAL LEG LIFT

**Starting Position:** Hand knee stand with right leg extended laterally and ankle flexed up toward lower leg.

**Action:** Slowly raise right leg up to hip level and slowly lower. Do not touch down to the floor. Repeat raising and lowering in succession. Repeat with left leg. Be sure legs are 'warmed-up' for this exercise!

# CHAPTER 13
## Program Planning

Earl Greer,

Captain, Armor

Program development guidelines
Muscle action and athletics
Principles of improvement
Selected exercise programs

An effective conditioning program requires proper planning. The selection of the best activities and exercises to develop a specific level of fitness or athletic competency mandates that the conditioning program be based on sound, scientific principles — **NOT INTUITION, SPECULATION, OR SUPERSTITION!**

## PROGRAM DEVELOPMENT GUIDELINES

The development of an effective conditioning program requires that an athlete answer three basic questions: What is my existing level of fitness?; What level of fitness do I want to achieve?; and How can I most effectively achieve my fitness goals? Honest, accurate responses to these questions will lead to a more productive personal conditioning program. The search for answers must be intelligently undertaken.

## SELF-EVALUATION

Relatively speaking, an athlete can evaluate his existing level of fitness by determining his fitness level on each of the basic aspects of fitness: cardiovascular fitness, endurance, strength, flexibility, and body composition. Each component of physical fitness can be tested by means of simple non-laboratory measures.

The most practical non-laboratory tests of **cardiovascular fitness** are Kenneth H. Cooper's (**Aerobics, The New Aerobics**) twelve-minute field test and modifications of what is known as a step test. In Cooper's 12 minute test, the athlete runs as far as he can in 12 minutes. In approximately ¼-mile yardage increments ranging from 1¾ miles for excellent to less than 1 mile for very poor, individuals are ranked as having an excellent, good, average, poor, or very poor level of cardiovascular fitness.

In the step test, the individual alternately steps up and down at a specific cadence on a bench (or similar device) which ranges in height from 12" to 20". The stepping goes on for a specific period of time and then the post-stepping heart rate is determined to estimate the athlete's adaptation to the demands placed on his cardiovascular system. For the most widely used step test (Harvard), the following scoring formula has been developed:

$$\text{Physical Efficiency Index} = \frac{\text{Duration of exercise in seconds X 100}}{5.5\text{X pulse count taken 1 to 1½ minutes after the stepping has finished}}$$

The following norms are usually arbitrarily used for evaluation:

Below 50 ............... Poor
50-80 .................. Average
Above 80 ............... Good

Regardless of what step test is used or normative system of evaluation is employed, all testing conditions should be standardized (time, bench height, cadence, length of the test, etc.). Pulse count is taken by placing the fingers either on the radial pulse (wrist) or on the carotid pulse (slight pressure to the left or right of the adam's apple).

**Muscle endurance** is measured by the individual working against a resistance representing less than his level of maximal strength. Isotonic (moving as opposed to static or isometric) endurance is usually tested by using the person's own body weight as the resistance. The most commonly employed endurance tests are pull-ups, chin-ups, push-ups, sit-ups and dips. Table 13-1 lists an arbitrary performance rating for these items.

| | Pull-ups | Chin-ups | Sit-ups | Push-ups (Bent Knee) | Dips (1 minute) |
|---|---|---|---|---|---|
| Excellent | 12+ | 14+ | 68+ | 50+ | 25+ |
| Good | 9-11 | 10-13 | 52-67 | 39-49 | 18-24 |
| Average | 6-8 | 6-9 | 36-51 | 25-38 | 9-17 |
| Poor | 3-5 | 3-5 | 29-35 | 12-24 | 4-8 |
| Very Poor | 0-2 | 0-2 | 0-28 | 0-11 | 0-3 |

Table 13-1. Normative scale for selective muscular endurance items. (Note: all scores are for men only; physical fitness testing "experts" have so **underestimated** the physical capabilities of athletically inclined women that the existing norms for women are apparently highly inaccurate).

Isotomic (moving) **strength** is tested by determining how much resistance (weight) a given muscle group can move through the full range of joint motion. Numerous mechanical- and operational differences between the various types of weight training equipment (Nautilus, Universal, and free weight) make it relatively **impossible** to compare strength measurements between the different types of equipment even though the same muscle group may be involved. Given the anatomical and neurological differences between individuals, a listing of the numerous norms for the various muscle groups would not be of value. One example of such an arbitrary norm is that an individual should be able to standing (military) press a weight equal to at least his own body weight in order to be considered above-average.

Flexibility is specific to a particular joint. As such, there is no single test which provides information about the flexibility of all the major joints of the body (see Chapter 1, Figures 1-1 and 1-2 for a complete listing of the normal range of motion for all of the body's major joints). An individual may be flexible in one area of the body and relatively inflexible in another. The flexibility requirements for effective performance in an activity vary not only from sport to sport but also from individual to individual. An example of a commonly used flexibility test is the trunk flexion test (Figure 13-1). Normally scored in inches (plus below the line, minus above the line), the average for college men is + 1″ and + 4″ for women.

There are no practical, relatively accurate non-laboratory methods of measuring **body composition.** Two tests which will provide an athlete with an estimation of body fat are the "pinch test" and the overweight index. The "pinch test" involves pinching the skin at selected areas of the body. Since body fat tends to be deposited in certain areas of the body (as opposed to being evenly distributed), the "pinch test" gives a rough indication of the amount of fat collected in a given area. To administer the "pinch test", the individual pinches his skin using his thumb and index finger. If the amount of skin between his fingers is greater than 1″, then the individual has an **excessive** amount of fat deposited in that area. One-half to one inch is considered to be too much but **moderate**; while less than a ½″ pinch of fat is judged to be an **acceptable** amount of fat. The five areas of the body which are usually measured are the triceps; the abdominal area surrounding the "bellybutton"; the lateral abdominal area (trunk); the inside of the upper thigh area; and the area at the bottom of the pectoralis (chest) muscles.

The overweight index (OWI) also provides an estimation of body fat. The formula for the OWI is:

OWI = 100 X bodyweight (kilograms) ÷ height (centimeters) — 100

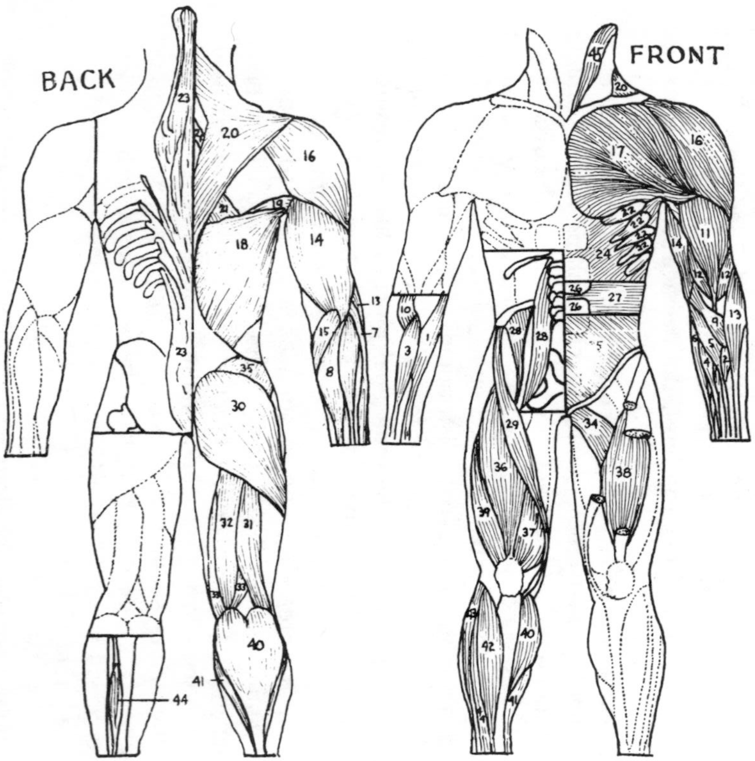

## DEFINITION OF ACTIONS

**FLEXION** — bending at a joint decreasing the angle. Does not apply to shoulder in this chart.

**EXTENSION** — straightening at a joint, opposite of flexion; not used for shoulder.

**ADDUCTION** — movement of a part toward the plane which splits the body into two equal halves, left and right.

**ABDUCTION** — opposite of adduction.

**ROTATION** — movement of a part around an axis.

**PRONATION** — rotation of forearm and hand to the palms-down position.

**SUPINATION** — rotation of forearm and hand to palms-up position; opposite of pronation.

**INVERSION** — twisting the foot outward at ankle.

**EVERSION** — bending the foot outward at ankle.

**ELEVATION** — raising of a part against gravity when in the standing position OR the same movement with the body in other than the standing position.

**DEPRESSION** — lowering of a part yielding to gravity when in the standing position OR the same movement with the body in other than the standing position; opposite of elevation.

Table 13-2. Definitions of muscle action. *

*Reprinted by permission of Cramer Products, Inc.

Figure 13-2. The musculature of the body. *
Refer to Table 13-3 for muscle identification.

*Reprinted by permission of Cramer Products, Inc.

Table 13-3. Muscle involvement in sports. *

| Muscle (corresponds to numbers in Figure 13-2) | Action Numbers in () indicate muscles which assist in action. | Sports In which greatest resistance is encountered. |
|---|---|---|
| 1. Flexor digitorium profundus<br>2. Flexor digitorium sublimus | Closes fingers | Any sport in which one grasps an opponent, partner or equipment, such as wrestling, hand to hand balancing, tennis, horizontal bar, ball bat, etc. |
| 3. Flexor pollicis longus | Flexes thumb | Tennis; throwing baseball; passing a football; handball; ring work; two handed pass in basketball; batting; golf swing. |
| 4. Palmaris longus<br>5. Flexor carpi radialis<br>6. Flexor carpi ulnaris | Flex wrist palmward and to both sides. (1, 2, 3, 7, 8) | |
| 7. Extensor carpi radialis longus and brevis<br>8. Extensor carpi ulnaris | Extends wrist | Backhand stroke in tennis and badminton; Olympic weight lifting; bait and fly casting. |
| 9. Pronator teres | Pronates forearm. | Tennis forehand; shot put; throwing a punch; throwing a baseball; passing a football. |
| 10. Supinator | Supination of forearm. (11) | Throwing a curve ball; batting; fencing thrust. |
| 11. Biceps brachii<br>12. Brachailis | Flexion of elbow. (9) | Ring work; rope climb; archery; pole vaulting; wrestling; back stroke in swimming. |
| 13. Brachioradialis | Strong elbow flexor with forearm pronated or partially pronated. | Rowing; cleaning a barbell; rope climbing. |
| 14. Triceps brachii<br>15. Anconeus | Extends the elbow. | Breast stroke; shot put; parallel bar work; vaulting; hand shivers in football; hand balancing; batting; pole vaulting; fencing thrust; passing both football or basketball; boxing. |

| # | Muscle | Action | Application |
|---|--------|--------|-------------|
| 16. | Deltoid. (For simplicity this muscle is divided into anterior and posterior fibers only.) | Anterior fibers—adduction, elevation, inward rotation of humerus. Posterior fibers — abduction, depression, outward rotation of humerus. | Hand balancing; canoeing; shot put; pole vaulting; tennis; archery; batting; fencing thrust; passing a football; tackling; breast stroke; back and crawl strokes; golf swing; handball. |
| 17. | Pectoralis major | (A) Forward elevation of humerus. (16, 19) (B) Adduction of humerus. (16, 19) (C) Inward rotation of humerus. (18, 19) | Tackling; crawl and back strokes; tennis; passing football; throwing a baseball; javelin; pole vaulting; wrestling; shot put; discus throw; straight arm lever position in gymnastics; punching. |
| 18. 19. | Latissimus dorsi / Teres major | Draws humerus down and backward. (16) Inward rotation of humerus. (16, 17) | Rope climb; canoe racing; ring work; rowing; batting; crawl, back, breast and butterfly strokes; pole vaulting; golf swing. |
| 20. | Trapezius | A. Tilts head back. (23) B. Elevates shoulder point. C. Adducts scapula. (21) | A. Wrestlers' bridge; B. Passing a football; cleaning a barbell; breast stroke. C. Archery; batting; breast stroke. |
| 21. | Rhomboids. Major & Minor | Adducts scapula. (20) | Tennis backhand; batting; back and breast strokes. |
| 22. | Serratus anterior | Abduction of scapula. | Shot put; discus throw; tennis; archery; tackling; crawl stroke; passing a basketball; passing a football; punching. |
| 23. | Spinea erector. (Also includes a number of smaller groups.) | A. Extension of spine. (20) B. Lateral flexion of spine. (20, 26, 27) C. Rotation of spine. | Discus and hammer throw; batting; golf swing; racing start in swimming; diving and tumbling; rowing; blocking in football. |
| 24. 25. 26. 27. | External oblique / Internal oblique / Rectus abdominus / Transversalis | Flexion of spine. Lateral flexion of spine. (23) Rotation of the spine. (23) Compression of abdomen. | The importance of this group of muscles in all sports, posture and general fitness and appearance cannot be overstated. |
| 28. | Illiopsoas | Flexion of trunk. (27) Flexion of thigh. (36) | Running; hurdling; pole vaulting; kicking a football; line play; flutter kick; pike and tuck positions in tumbling and diving. |
| 29. | Sartorius | Flexion of femur. (39) Flexion of knee. Rotates femur outward. | Tumbling and diving. |

| Muscle | Action | Activity |
|---|---|---|
| 30. Gluteus maximus | Extends femur. (31, 32, 33) Outward rotation of femur. (31) | Skiing; shot put; running; quick starts in track; all jumping and skipping; line play; skating; swimming start; changing direction while running. |
| 31. Biceps Femoris | Extension of femur. (30) Flexion of knee. (40) Outward rotation of femur. (30) | Skiing; skating; quick starts in track and swimming; hurdling; line play; all jumping. |
| 32. Semitendenosus 33. Semimembranosus | Flexion of knee. (40) Flexion of femur. (30) Inward rotation of femur. | |
| 34. Adductor magnus | Adduction of femur and outward rotation during adduction. | Skiing; skating; frog kick; broken field running; bareback horseback riding. |
| 35. Gluteus medius | Abduction of femur. (Essential for spring) | Hurdling; fencing; frog kick; shot put; running; line play; skating. |
| 36. Rectus femoris | Flexion of femur. (28) Extension of knee. | Skiing; skating; quick starts; all jumping; kick in football or soccer; flutter kick; frog kick; water skiing; diving; trampoline and tumbling; bicycling; catching in baseball. |
| 37. Vastus internus 38. Vastus intermedius 39. Vastus externus | Extension of knee. | |
| 40. Gastrocnemius | Extension of foot. (44) (when knee is almost straight) | Quick starts in track; swimming; basketball; football; skating; all jumping; skiing. |
| 41. Soleus | Extension of foot. (when knee is bent) | |
| 42. Tibialis anterior | Flexes foot and inverts it. | Changing direction while running; skating; skiing. |
| 43. Peroneus longus | Extension of foot. (40, 41, 44) Eversion of foot. | Skating turns; changing direction while running. |
| 44. Flexor hallucis longus | Flexion of big toe. Extension of ankle. | Running; all jumping; racing starts. |
| 45. Sternomastoid | Tucking of chin. Rotation of head. Raises sternum in deep breathing. | Crawl stroke; tucking chin in wrestling, football, boxing; distance running (breathing). |

*Reprinted by permission of Cramer Products, Inc.

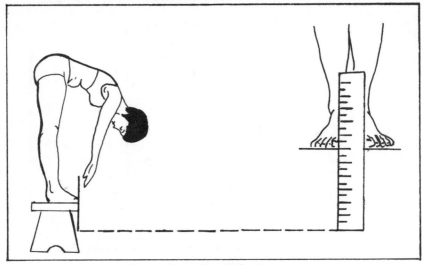

Figure 13-1. Trunk flexion test.

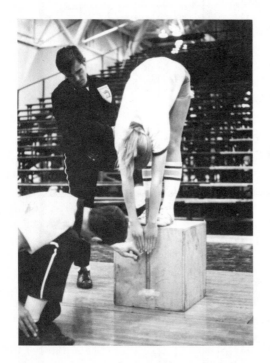

"Project 60" subject from a USMA research project performing the trunk flexion test.

On the OWI, a score in excess of 110 represents obesity.

## ESTABLISH OBJECTIVES

Given an evaluation of the athlete's level of fitness, the next step is to establish realistic goals for the conditioning program. The program objectives should be based on at least three factors: an accurate assessment of the athlete's existing level of fitness; a reasonable determination of what degree of personal fitness improvement can be achieved within existing time, equipment, and environmental considerations; and a realistic evaluation of the fitness requirements for the sport in which the athlete is interested.

## SELECT PROGRAM

Program selection is based on a number of factors: personal goals, facilities and equipment, time, environmental conditions, personal attitudes, and existing level of fitness. Whatever exercise regimen is eventually adopted, the athlete should periodically re-evaluate his level of progress in order to determine whether or not program goals are being met and whether or not an adjustment in the conditioning program is required.

### MUSCLE ACTION AND ATHLETICS

Participation in any athletic activity normally involves almost every major muscle in the body. The actual involvement of the various muscle groups, however, varies from activity to activity. Athletes and coaches who are interested in developing effective conditioning programs should analyze their sports in order to determine which muscles are involved. Once the important muscles are identified, the exercise program can be tailored to the activity's developmental needs. Figure 13-2 and Tables 13-2 and 13-3 provide an inclusive listing of muscles, muscle actions, and the sports in which the muscles are involved.

### PRINCIPLES OF IMPROVEMENT

Regardless of which conditioning program the athlete selects, the program **must** be based on certain specific principles if fitness improvement is to be maximized. For each aspect of fitness, there are selected rules-of-thumb which should be followed. Since there are a number of differences between individuals the **exact** principles and guidelines vary slightly from individual to individual.

## CARDIOVASCULAR FITNESS

1. Substantial **demand** must be placed on the cardiovascular system. In general, a heart rate of 140-160 beats per minute for 10-15 minutes should be achieved 4 to 5 times per week.

2. As much of the body's **total musculature** as possible should be involved in the activity.

3. The activity must be at a level of **intensity** which will produce an appropriate demand on the cardiovascular system. Intense, but not too intense.

4. The activity should be engaged in for a period of **duration** long enough to generate improvement.

5. The activity should be **regular.** Four to five times a week is a guideline for developing a conditioning base. Once an adequate level of cardiovascular fitness is achieved, it may be maintained with slightly fewer weekly workouts.

## STRENGTH

1. A **demand** must be placed on the muscles the athlete wishes to strengthen.

2. The position for initiating the greatest force is one in which the muscle is **stretched** slightly.

3. Each exercise should be performed through the **full range of movement.**

4. A workout program should be performed three days a week with **adequate rest** (48-72 hours) between individual workouts.

5. Whenever possible, a workout program should include **negative-only** training.

## MUSCULAR ENDURANCE

1. A **demand** to persist for an extended period of time must be placed on the muscles the athlete wishes to improve.

2. At a given load, **higher levels of strength** generally provide for greater levels of muscular endurance.

3. Muscular endurance at a given load is generally related not directly to an individual's level of strength but to a **specific percentage** of his ability to generate maximum force.

## FLEXIBILITY

1. A **demand** for full extension, flexion, or both must be placed on the joint.

2. **Stretch slowly and smoothly.**

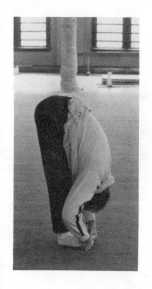 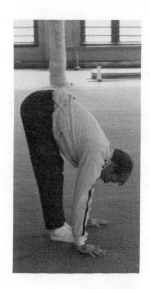 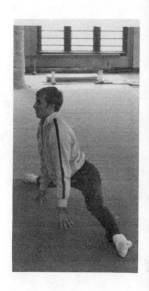

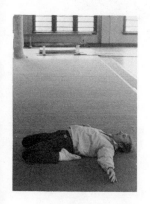 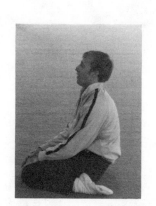 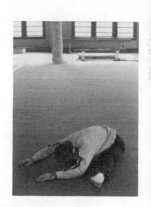

One-person flexibility exercises.

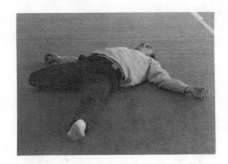
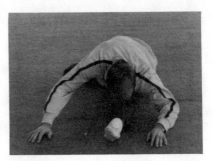

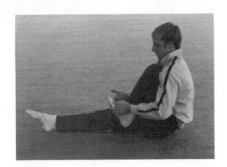
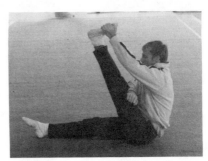

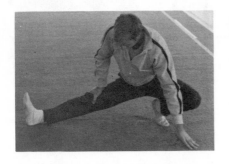
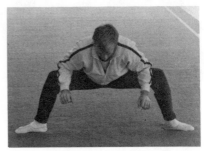

One-person flexibility exercises.

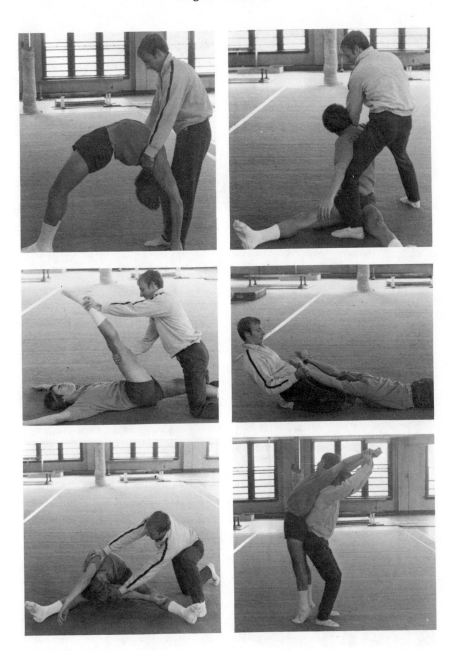

Two-person flexibility exercises.

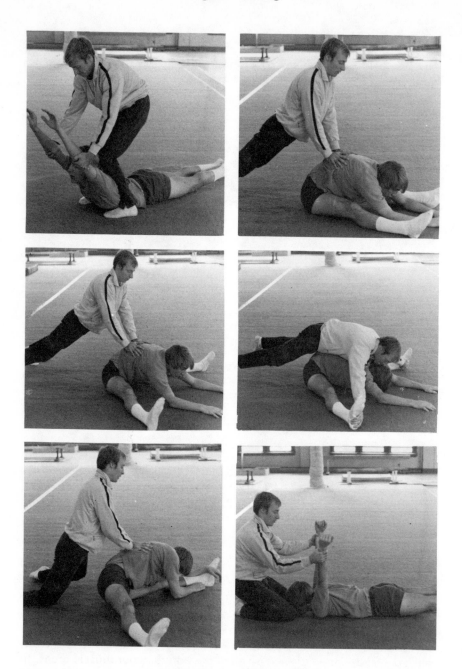

Two-person flexibility exercises.

3. **Practice regularly.**
4. **Distributed** (several sessions at different times) flexibility exercising is a better method for developing flexibility than **massed** (once a day) practice.

## BODY COMPOSITION

1. The diet must be **nutritionally sound.**
2. Eat the **proper amount** of food.
3. Eat **regularly.**
4. **Exercise** regularly.
5. Avoid **empty calories.**

## SELECTED EXERCISE PROGRAMS
### AEROBICS

"Aerobics" is a widely proclaimed program developed by Dr. Kenneth H. Cooper. Through laboratory testing, Cooper measured the oxygen consumption cost (amount used) of various activities performed at various intensities (rates of speed, length of time) and arbitrarily assigned these calculations an equivalent "point" value. The point values assigned to the various activities represent perceived oxygen consumption. The higher the oxygen use, the more points awarded under Cooper's system. Depending on his arbitrary fitness category (based on Cooper's 12-minute run—see the section in this Chapter on evaluating cardiovascular fitness), an individual attempts to achieve a predetermined number of "points" per week. Table 13-4 lists the point system which USMA employs in its aerobics course. Based on Cooper's **New Aerobics,** the point values have been adjusted for clarity and simplicity and to reflect the high level of fitness of the Corps of Cadets.

### CALISTHENICS (U.S. ARMY CONDITIONING DRILL)

Achieveing and maintaining an adequate level of physical fitness in every soldier is a major goal of the United States Army. To help accomplish this objective, most Army commanders require that their soldiers engage in a program of regular, progressive exercise. In most instances, the foundation of such a program is regular participation in U.S. Army conditioning drills 1, 2, and 3 (Figure 13-3). Containing seven exercises, each drill is designed to exercise **all** of the body's major muscle areas. In general, each set of exercises can be completed in approximately 15 minutes and can serve as an excellent warm-up program for more rigorous exercise.

## Table 13-4. Point system used in the USMA aerobics program.

- To receive a passing grade in the course, a cadet must earn a maximum of 50 points per week.
- To compute the point totals for activities which are not listed, select the activity closest in nature to the unlisted activity (e.g. soccer and team handball) and use the point totals for that activity.

1. Activity* (distance in a prescribed time)

|  | Distance | Time | Point Value |
|---|---|---|---|
| a. Running | 1.0 miles | 9:00 | 4 |
|  | 1.0 miles | 8:00 | 5 |
|  | 1.0 miles | 7:00 | 6 |
| 1.0 miles | 6:00 | 7 | |
|  |  |  |  |
| b. Swimming | 100 yds. | 2:30 | 1 |
| (freestyle) | 100 yds. | 2:30 | 2 |
|  | 100 yds. | 1:30 | 3 |

*To compute the point value for longer distances, multiply by a factor of 1 mile for running and 100 yds. for swimming. For example, a 2-mile run performed in a time of less than 18 minutes earns the runner 8 pts. A 200-yard swim in less than 5 minutes earns the swimmer 2 points.

2. Activity** (participate for a prescribed length of time)

|  | Length of time | Point Value |
|---|---|---|
| a. Handball-Racquetball-Squash-Basketball | 30 min. | 5 |
|  | 60 min. | 10 |
| b. Soccer-Rugby-Lacrosse Flickerball | 30 min. | 9 |
|  | 60 min. | 18 |
| c. Skiing (water or snow) | 30 min. | 3 |
|  | 60 min. | 6 |
| d. Tennis (singles) | 30 min. | 2.5 |
|  | 60 min. | 5 |
| e. USMA Circuit | Time — 15 minutes or less | |

| Difficulty Level | Points |
|---|---|
| Beginner | 7 |
| Average | 8 |
| Good | 9 |
| Excellent | 10 |
| Superior | 12 |

**To compare the point value for a longer amount of time, multiply by a factor of either 30 minutes or 60 minutes.

# CONDITIONING DRILL

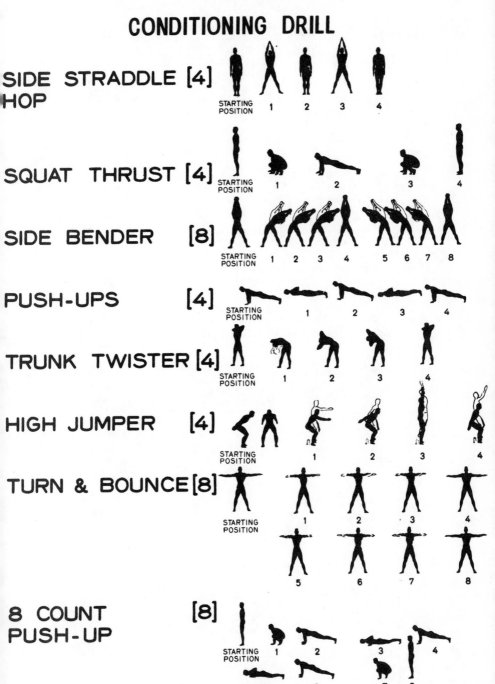

Figure 13-3. U.S. Army Conditioning Drill #1.

## Table 13-5. An interval training program designed to improve an individual's 2-mile run time.

**KEY**

Running time per interval:
- (110)  3 sec slower than 110 from a standing start.
- (220)  5 sec slower than 220 from a standing start.
- (440)  The average 440 time for the best mile run time.
- (880)  4 sec slower than twice the average 440 time for the best mile run time.

Resting time between intervals:
  For the enclosed program, a specific rest time between intervals is suggested. For example, (1:3) means that the individual should rest between intervals for an amount equal to three times the amount of time taken to run the interval.

Resting time between sets:
  The rest time between sets should be sufficient to enable the pulse rate of the individual to go down to a maximum of 150 beats per minute.

**FIRST WEEK**

| Day | | Number of reps | | Length of interval | Rest Period |
|---|---|---|---|---|---|
| 1 | Set 1 | 5 | x | 220 | (1:3) |
|   | Set 2 | 8 | x | 110 | (1:3) |
| 2 | Set 1 | 2 | x | 440 | (1:3) |
|   | Set 2 | 8 | x | 110 | (1:3) |
| 3 | Set 1 | 2 | x | 440 | (1:3) |
|   | Set 2 | 6 | x | 220 | (1:3) |
| 4 | Set 1 | 1 | x | 880 | |
|   | Set 2 | 6 | x | 220 | (1:3) |
| 5 | 2 mile rune (75% effort) | | | | |

**SECOND WEEK**

| Day | | Number of reps | | Length of interval | Rest Period |
|---|---|---|---|---|---|
| 1 | Set 1 | 2 | x | 880 | (1:3) |
|   | Set 2 | 2 | x | 440 | (1:3) |
| 2 | Set 1 | 6 | x | 440 | (1:3) |
| 3 | Set 1 | 3 | x | 880 | (1:3) |
|   | Set 2 | 4 | x | 110 | (1:3) |
| 4 | Set 1 | 2 | x | 1-mile run | (1:3) |
|   | at an 80% effort | | | | |
| 5 | 2 mile run (75% effort) | | | | |

**THIRD WEEK**

| Day | | Number of reps | of interval | Length Period | Rest |
|---|---|---|---|---|---|
| 1 | Set 1 | 8 | x | 110 | (1:2) |
| 2 | Set 1 | 1 | x | 110 | (1:1) |
|   | Set 2 | 4 | x | 220 | (1:2) |
|   | Set 3 | 2 | x | 880 | (1:2) |
| 3 | Set 1 | 6 | x | 110 | (1:2) |
|   | Set 2 | 1 | x | 880 | (3 min.) |
|   | Set 3 | 4 | x | 110 | (1:2) |
|   | Set 4 | 2 | x | 440 | (1:3) |
| 4 | 2 mile run (75% effort) | | | | |
| 5 | 2 mile run (maximum effort) | | | | |

**FOURTH WEEK**

| Day | | Number of reps | | Length of interval | Rest Period |
|---|---|---|---|---|---|
| 1 | Set 1 | 2 | x | 220 | (1:2) |
|   | Set 2 | 2 | x | 440 | (1:3) |
|   | Set 3 | 2 | x | 880 | (1:3) |

## CIRCUIT TRAINING

Circuit training is a method of conditioning that generally is geared towards the development of all-around fitness. The term "circuit" refers to a number of specifically selected exercises arranged about a given area. Each exercise in a circuit is referred to as a station. Under this arrangement, the athlete progresses from one station to another, performing a specific amount of work at each station until the entire circuit has been completed. The time the individual takes to complete the circuit is usually recorded. Progression on the circuit is identified by increasing the work required at each station, decreasing the amount of time required to complete the circuit, or both.

As a program of conditioning, circuit training has numerous desireable characteristics. It is extremely adaptable to a number of varying situations. For example, the circuit can be adapted for a variety of purposes, time limitations, size of groups, etc. Circuit training provides an opportunity for individual **progression.** The individual works at his own rate. His degree of improvements depends almost entirely on his own initiative and efforts. The time-factor in circuit training serves both as an excellent **built-in motivator** and as a reasonably accurate **self-testing measure.** The individual is encouraged to push himself to perform better by lowering his time to complete the circuit.

## INTERVAL TRAINING

Interval training is a method of exercising in which several variables are manipulated in order to produce a training effect: the amount of time an athlete engages in the program on any particular day; the length of the run (distance) or the number of repeitions of an exercise performed; the rate or level of intensity of a particular interval; and the amount of rest between intervals.

In general, interval training is normally used to develop either cardiovascular fitness or muscular endurance. As an exercise technique, however, interval training can be applied to numerous forms of conditioning because all forms of exercise involve work and rest. Not only can the work-rest periods be used for progression, but the amount and kind of work can be varied as well. Table 13-5 outlines an example of an interval training program used at West Point to improve 2-mile run time.

## WEIGHT TRAINING*
*Refer to Chapters 3-6.

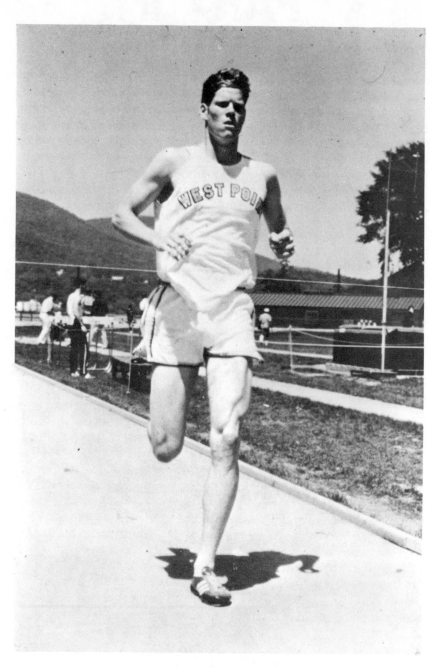

Curt Alitz (Class of 1978), the greatest runner in USMA's history.

# PART II

## CONDITIONING PROGRAMS
### for
## SELECTED SPORTS

| | |
|---|---|
| Baseball | Lacrosse |
| Basketball | Racquetball |
| Bowling | Rugby |
| Boxing | Skiing |
| Field Hockey | Soccer |
| Football | Swimming |
| Golf | Team Handball |
| Gymnastics | Tennis |
| Handball | Track and Field |
| Ice Hockey | Volleyball |
| Judo | Wrestling |

## INTRODUCTION TO PART II

Given the information presented in Part I of this book (Chapters 1-13), it is apparent that success for any individual who participates in sports and athletics is dependent upon a variety of factors. Improvement in each of these components can be achieved through a combination of hard work, adherence to scientific principles, and personal dedication.

Part II of this book presents specific conditioning programs for twenty-two separate sports. Although the limitations inherent in prescribing a "cook-book" program for an activity are recognized, certain benefits can be gained from such programs. Relative to an athlete's situation, a "reasonable" starting point is identified; a comprehensive "total conditioning" plan is presented; and an overview of the sport serves as a basis for self-evaluation and program adjustment.

The emphasis in Part II is on muscular development for specific sports. In selected chapters, drills to develop other aspects of fitness required for sports participation are also presented. For all sports, guidelines for following a conditioning program both during the off-season and the in-season are discussed. In general, the in-season program is usually a less-frequent (twice-a-week instead of 3x) and less-extensive (fewer exercises) application of the off-season program.

Because a listing of the drills and techniques used to develop specific motor abilities for any given sport would be an endless task, the following general principles for improving selected motor abilities are recommended:

### AGILITY

1. Practice the activity.
2. Place a demand upon the systems involved.
3. Accuracy and speed should be combined in equal amounts.
4. Distributed (versus massed) practice provides the optimum level of improvement.
5. Repetition is essential.
6. Don't push past the point of fatigue.

### BALANCE

1. Place a demand on the systems involved.
2. Mental practice is usually beneficial.
3. Whenever necessary, sacrifice speed for accuracy.
4. Repetition is essential.
5. Distributed (versus massed) practice is best.
6. Overload the senses (e.g. the individual closes his eyes)
7. Try to improve balance in as many different body positions and as many kinds of movement as possible.

## COORDINATION

1. Practice the activity **accurately**! Accuracy is more important than speed.
2. Place a demand on the systems involved.
3. Distributed (versus massed) practice is best.
4. Repetition is essential.
5. Don't practice past the point of neuromuscular fatigue.

## POWER

1. Develop the involved musculature (weight training).
2. Develop the neuromuscular coordination involved (practice the movement).
3. The rate of working should be increased (increase the speed of movement).
4. The force of application should be increased (exert greater explosive movement).

## REACTION TIME

(reaction time is the ability to react to a certain stimulus; it is frequently referred to as "quickness")

1. Place a demand on systems involved.
2. Regular practice is required.
3. To a certain extent, the development of "quickness" is inhibited by specific genetic limitations.

## SPEED

1. Place a demand on the specific movement.
2. Practice the movement involved.
3. Develop the involved musculature (weight training).
4. Overloading the body movements involved in speed (e.g. by wearing leg or ankle weights) is of "doubtful" value.

For each sport, the athlete should identify the motor abilities required for successful participation in that activity and should select drills based upon the aforementioned "improvement principles" to develop those motor abilities.

# CHAPTER 14
## Baseball

Some individuals claim that baseball demands more of an athlete's all-around natural ability than any other sport. It is a sport that requires a high level of hand-eye coordination, quickness with both hands and feet, power and endurance. Professional ball players are continually practicing and playing to keep their skills as sharp as possible. During the course of a season they rarely have time to follow a regular workout schedule. During the off-season and pre-season, however, everything is usually quite different. Workouts are generally undertaken on a regular basis.

Amateur baseball is obviously quite different from professional baseball, not only because of the skill level, but because of the level of physical condition of the participant. The amateur baseball player who plays a few nights a week or just on weekends typically feels that this amount of exercise is adequate to keep him in shape and keep his skills sharp. The typical pre-season and off-season workouts for non-professional athletes consist of nothing more than a pickup game of basketball or some other type of informal session. Then these individual wonder why they pull muscles running or injure their arms and shoulders throwing once the baseball season commences.

For the amateur ballplayer to avoid these injuries and improve his performance, he should exercise year round. The athlete should devote approximately 30 minutes at least 3-4 times a week to a well-planned workout schedule.

Obviously nothing can replace the actual practice of throwing, hitting, fielding, and running. These require certain motor abilities that must be practiced frequently if they are to be developed, maintained and improved upon. To help improve his baseball performance, the athlete should concentrate on improving his level of muscular development. For example, by strengthening the muscles used to throw, the athlete can minimize elbow and shoulder injuries and improve his level of endurance. As a result, the athlete can throw relatively hard for a longer period of time. Through a muscular development program, the base runner can improve his body speed, substantially decrease the possibility of incurring a serious leg injury, and increase his level of overall quickness. The hitter can not only increase his bat speed which is the most fundamental aspect of successful hitting, but also add more power

*The editor is grateful to David Yates for his assistance in writing this chapter.

to his swing. All of these things can be achieved if an athlete is willing to devote approximately 30 minutes three or four times a week. It is a relatively small sacrifice to achieve skill improvement.

Table 14-1. Baseball overview.

| BASIC SKILLS | MUSCLES INVOLVED |
|---|---|
| 1. Hitting | Hips, lead arm triceps, wrist, shoulders |
| 2. Running | Legs, buttocks |
| 3. Throwing | Hips, legs, back, shoulder, girdle, elbow, wrist |

PROBLEM AREAS:

Knees, ankles
Shoulders
Elbows
Muscle fatigue

AREAS TO EMPHASIZE:

- grip for bat control—develop the forearm flexors

- upper back (latissimus dorsi)—primary muscle in the upper body used for throwing

- elbow—develop the muscles of the upper arm (biceps-triceps) to minimize the possibility of hyperextending or violently jamming of the elbow joint while throwing

## Table 14-2. Off-season Baseball Nautilus Workout Program

| EXERCISE (in order) | PRIMARY MUSCLES DEVELOPED | SPECIFIC SKILLS INVOLVED |
|---|---|---|
| 1. Hip and Back* | Buttocks, lower back | Running, hitting, throwing |
| 2. Leg Extension | Quadriceps | Running, throwing, hitting |
| 3. Leg Press* | Buttocks, quadriceps | Running, hitting, throwing |
| 4. Leg Curl* | Hamstrings | Running, hitting, throwing |
| 5. Double Shoulder* (seated press) | Deltoids | Throwing, hitting |
| 7.¹Pullover* | Latissimus dorsi | Throwing, hitting |
| 8. Chin-ups* | Latissimus dorsi, biceps, forearm flexors | Throwing, hitting (grip) |
| 9. Dips* | Pectorals, deltoids, triceps | Throwing, hitting (extension of lead arm tricep at impact) |
| 10. Biceps Curls | Biceps | Throwing (breaking ball) assist in pronating the arm |
| 11. Wrist Curls* | Forearm flexors | Throwing, hitting |

- Perform 1 set of 8 to 12 reps of each exercise

- Take no more than 60 seconds to perform each set

- Rest no more than 30 seconds between each set

- To determine *total workout time*: multiply # of workouts by 1½ minutes, then subtract 30 seconds from total

*In-season only

## Table 14-3. Off-season Baseball Universal Workout Program

| EXERCISE (in order) | PRIMARY MUSCLES DEVELOPED | SPECIFIC SKILLS INVOLVED |
|---|---|---|
| 1. Leg Press* | Buttocks, quadriceps | Running, throwing, hitting |
| 2. Leg Extension* | Quadriceps | Running, throwing, hitting |
| 3. Leg Curl* | Hamstrings | Running, throwing, hitting |
| 4. Bench Press* | Pectorals, deltoids, triceps | Throwing, hitting |
| 5. Chin-ups* | Latissimus dorsi, biceps | Throwing, hitting, (grip) |
| 6. Seated Press | Deltoids, triceps | Throwing, hitting |
| 7. Lat Pulldown | Latissimus dorsi, biceps | Throwing, hitting |
| 8. Triceps Extension* | Triceps | Throwing, hitting, extension of lead arm tricep at impact |
| 9. Biceps Curl* | Biceps | Throwing (breaking ball) assist in pronating the arm |
| 10. Wrist Curl* | Forearm flexors | Throwing, hitting |

- Perform 1 set of 8 to 12 reps of each exercise

- Take no more than 60 seconds to perform each set

- Rest no more than 30 seconds between each set

- To determine *total workout time:* multiply # of workouts by 1½ minutes, then subtract 30 seconds from total.

*In-season only

## Table 14-4. An off-season conditioning program for baseball pitchers.*

Outlined below is an off-season, light weight-lifting program designed to strengthen the arm, shoulder and latissimus dorsi muscles. **This program will not make you muscle-bound.** Its primary effect will be to:

1) decrease the possibility of developing a sore arm
2) increase your endurance over the course of the season

The weight is a 10 or 12 lb. dumbbell and it remains constant. **Do not increase the weight.**

A set consists of five exercises. Do three sets a day, every other day. Never do them two days in a row.

Start with **5** repetitions of each exercise. Rest between each of the three sets of about 5 minutes. Swing a bat or stretch your arms to keep them loose. Then go back and do another set. The whole program should take only a half hour to 45 minutes per day.

Do the three sets of 5 repetitions for 2-3 weeks. After three weeks, you may go to 7 repetitions, after five weeks, you may go to 10 repetitions, after eight weeks, you may go to 12 repetitions, after 10 weeks, you may go to 15 repetitions and after 12 weeks you may go to 20 repetitions. When you have reached the 20 repetitions, maintain this level to the start of Spring Training.

Described below are the five exercises which must be done with both arms — you cannot overdevelop one side:

1. With dumbbell in hand, raise the arm with elbow bent forward to approximately eye level so that the thumb is facing the floor and back of hand is facing the ceiling. Extend forearm up towards ceiling — then back down. Do not let the weight drop — let it down, slowly. Repeat 5 times. Do same with other arm.

2. Arm straight down at side, raise weight to the side (keeping arm stiff — do not bend elbow) shoulder high and back down again. Repeat five times. Do same on other side.

3. Arm in hanging position, palm facing to the rear, extend arm to the front, shoulder high, up in front of your eyes. Do not swing weight, bring down to stop when you come down with it. Repeat five times. Do same on other side.

4. Arm in hanging position (same as above), extend arm to the rear. Naturally, you will not be able to bring arm shoulder high but go as far as you can. Bring back to hanging position. Do not swing weight. Repeat five times. Do same on other side.

5. Raise arm, bending elbow so that fist is shoulder high and palm is facing ceiling. Extend straight up and then return to original position. Repeat five times. Do same on other side.

*The aforementioned program was enclosed in a letter to the editor of this book from N.Y. Mets' pitcher Tom Seaver — one of the greatest players of all time. Seaver was responding to a request for his personal off-season conditioning program.

Table 14-5. University of Delaware's Baseball Program "Go" Routine

---

• A combination of strength and flexibility exercises. Learn to execute each item **correctly** for maximum benefit to you personally.

• This is a highly individualized program and should be done by each player **even on non-practice days.** Your consistency in pushing this phase of your daily workout could make the difference in **your overall success!!!!**

• **Pitchers:** In addition to the "Go" Routine and Running, the athlete should do daily **pick-ups!!!** NO EXCEPTIONS UNLESS THE ATHLETE FIRST checks with the coaches. Start with 50 daily for the first week, 75 for the second and increase by increments of 25 per week.

• This program should be done **everyday** during the preseason and regular season including game dates. The "Go" routine has helped to reduce the number of sore arms and muscle pulls that a player will incur during the course of a season.

KEY POINTS
1. **Do not bounce on any stretch item.**
2. Each stretch repetition must be held for minimum of three (3) seconds or as directed.
3. **Think** relaxation as you move through items.
4. Most Important: In order to gain maximum benefit from these items, the correct body position must be learned and consistently used in execution.
5. The individual working by himself should be able to go through the entire program in 10 minutes or less.

I. WARM-UPS
   1. Jog in place.
   2. Two foot jump or toe bounce
   3. Shoulders
      Side benders — (Hand over head)
      Standing back arch — (Hands over head)
      Chest expansion — (Hands behind back)
   4. Hip circles (alternate directions)
   5. Pike stand — hands behind knees
   6. Wide straddle stand
   7. Standing groin stretch (on heel)
   8. Standing leg kicks
   9. Quads stretch
  10. Hurdler's stretch
  11. Deep pike/straddle lying (alternate)
  12. Inverted back arch

II. WARM-DOWNS
   1. Inverted arch walk
   2. 20 sit-ups
   3. Leg scissors (sitting)
   4. 20 push-ups
   5. Ankle walk on inside and outside of ankles

III. RUNNING
   On alternate days,
   **sprints** and **one mile run.**

---

# CHAPTER 15
## Basketball

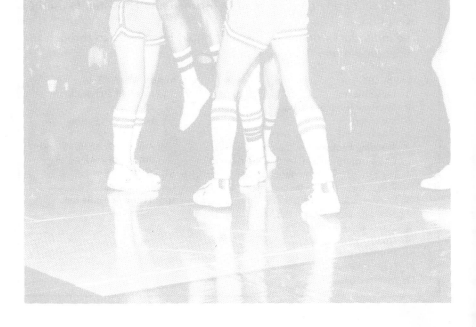

In recent years, there has been increasing emphasis on basketball players who can run faster, jump higher, and play more aggressively. As a result, there has been a concommitant increase in the demand for effective conditioning programs for basketball players at all levels— secondary school, intercollegiate, professional, and recreational-free time, Naturally, conditioning at each level should be geared both to the individual and to the desired level of competency.

Proper conditioning for basketball involves, not only improvement in the athlete's level of muscular development, but also substantial time devoted to increasing cardiovascular fitness and flexibility. For general guidelines on how to effectively develop these components of fitness, the athlete should refer to Part I of this text. Particular attention should be given to an extension program of interval training.

The basketball player should remember that proper conditioning is a **year-round** responsibility. Because the typical basketball season is several months long, there is a tendency to overlook the necessity for some type of in-season, "fitness-maintenance" program. On the contrary, a well-planned in-season conditioning program can diminish both the onslaught of muscular fatigue and the chances of a player suffering a serious injury.

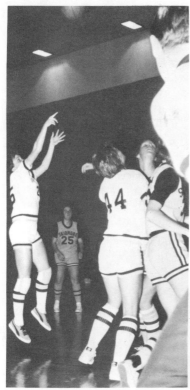

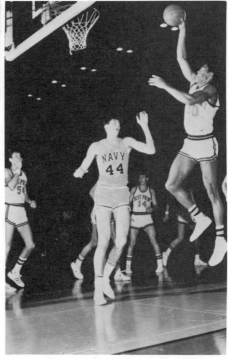

Basketball is an extremely popular sport for both men and women.

## Table 15-1. Basketball overview

| BASIC SKILLS | MUSCLES INVOLVED |
|---|---|
| 1. Jumping | Buttocks, quadriceps, hamstrings |
| 2. Throwing | Latissimus dorsi, deltoids, pectorals, triceps |
| 4. Dribbling | Hand-wrist flexors |

PROBLEM AREAS:

Knees, ankles
Shoulders
Aerobic capacity (stamina)
Muscle fatigue

AREAS TO EMPHASIZE:

- grip for holding on to the ball—develop the forearm flexors and the biceps to increase grip strength for holding on to the ball, pulling it away from an opponent, etc.

- shooting muscles—develop muscles used in shooting so that shooting capability will not be affected by muscular fatigue.

- knee—strengthen the knee to decrease its susceptibility to injury.

## Table 15-2. Off-season Basketball Nautilus Workout Program

| EXERCISE (in order) | PRIMARY MUSCLES DEVELOPED | SPECIFIC SKILLS INVOLVED (each exercise helps to improve rebounding and ball control) |
|---|---|---|
| 1. Hip and Back* | Buttocks | Rebounding, running |
| 2. Leg Extension | Quadriceps | Jumping, running |
| 3. Leg Press* | Buttocks, quadriceps | Jumping, running |
| 4. Leg Curl* | Hamstrings | Running forward and backward |
| 5. Double Shoulder* (lateral raise) | Deltoids | Shooting |
| 6. Double Shoulder* | Deltoids, triceps | Shooting, passing |
| 7. Pullover* | Latissimus dorsi | Throwing, battling for a rebound |
| 8. Chin-up | Latissimus dorsi, biceps | Throwing, pulling a ball away from an opponent |
| 9. Infi-bench | Pectorals, deltoids, | Shooting, throwing, passing |
| 10. Biceps Curl* | Biceps | Pulling a ball away from an opponent while rebounding |
| 11. Wrist Curl* | Forearm flexors | Shooting, gripping, wrist control, passing |
| 12. Squeeze rubber ball | Hand flexors | Shooting, dribbling |

- Perform 1 set of 8 to 12 reps of each exercise

- Take no more than 60 seconds to perform each set

- *: Rest no more than 30 seconds between each set

- To determine *total workout time:* multiply # of workouts by 1½ minutes, then subtract 30 seconds from total

*In-season only

## Table 15-3. Off-season Basketball Universal Workout Program

| EXERCISE (in order) | PRIMARY MUSCLES DEVELOPED | SPECIFIC SKILLS INVOLVED (each exercise helps to improve rebounding and ball control) |
|---|---|---|
| 1. Leg Press* | Buttocks, quadriceps | Running, Jumping |
| 2. Leg Extension | Quadriceps | Running, jumping |
| 3. Leg Curl* | Hamstrings | Running forward and backwards |
| 4. Bench Press* | Pectorals, deltoids, triceps | Throwing, shooting, passing |
| 5. Chin-ups* | Latissimus dorsi, biceps | Throwing, pulling a ball away from an opponent |
| 6. Seated Press | Deltoids, triceps | Shooting, passing |
| 7. Lat Pulldown | Latissimus dorsi, biceps | Throwing, pulling a ball away from an opponent |
| 8. Triceps extension* | Triceps | Shooting, passing |
| 9. Biceps Curls* | Biceps | Pulling a ball away from an opponent |
| 10. Wrist Curl* | Forearm flexors | Shooting, gripping, wrist control, passing |
| 11. Rubber Ball Squeeze* | Hand flexors | Dribbling, shooting |

- Perform 1 set of 8 to 12 reps of each exercise

- Take no more than 60 seconds to perform each set

- Rest no more than 30 seconds between each set

- To determine *total workout time:* multiply # of workouts by 1½ minutes, then subtract 30 seconds from total

*In-season only

Table 15-4. Sample of a circuit for basketball conditioning.

| Station 1 | Station 2 | Station 3 | Station 4 |
|-----------|-----------|-----------|-----------|
| **Agility Drill** | **Rebound Release** | **Run Stairs** | **Bench Jump** |
| Station 8 | Station 7 | Station 6 | Station 5 |
| WHISTLE **Reverse Drill** | **Board Tipping** | **Shuffle Drill** | **Rope Skipping** |

KEY

**Agility Drill** — From the free throw line, the athlete faces the backboard, shuffles to the corner, sprints to the key, and back pedals to the end line. Perform 6 times.

**Rebound Release Drill** — From the free throw line, the athlete throws the ball against the board, rebounds, and releases to an outlet man; then he sprints back to the free throw line, takes a pass from the release man, re-passes to the release man, re-passes to the release man, and in turn is given the ball back from the release man and then takes a lay-up.

**Run Stairs** — Run 10 sets of stairs; vigorously while running up the stairs, moderately while going down the stairs.

**Bench Jump** — Athlete stands parallel to a bench 12"-18" high, jumps over and back quickly for as many repetitions as possible.

**Rope Skipping** — Athlete jumps rope, alternating feet for 5 minutes

**Shuffle Drill** — Athlete responds to directional signals from another individual, shuffles side to side and back and forth; movement is kept constant for 2 minutes.

**Board Tipping** — Athlete tips the ball against the backboard using one hand for as long as possible.

**Whistle Reverse Drill** — On the sound of the whistle, athlete runs as fast as he can in a straight line; when the whistle sounds again, the athlete reverses himself as quickly as possible; repeat 10 times.

# CHAPTER 16
## Bowling

Bowling is an activity which requires a high level of precision and accuracy. The bowler must discipline the body to repeat exactly the controlled approach and smooth pendulum-motion of the delivery. Bowling, as a general rule, does not requir an extraordinate level of muscular development. Muscular fatigue, however, can have an adverse affect on the consistency and accuracy of a bowler's delivery. The best method for eliminating or reducing such fatigue is weight training.

A properly-planned muscular development program can enable the "league" bowler to sustain his precision and accuracy for a longer period of time. Since there is no off-season for the "average" bowler, a conditioning program should be employed 2 or 3 times a week depending on the athlete's existing level of fitness and amount of available time.

---

Table 16-1. Bowling overview

| BASIC SKILLS | MUSCLES INVOLVED |
|---|---|
| 1. Approach | Quadriceps, hamstrings, buttocks |
| 2. Delivery of the ball (backswing and release) | Deltoids, latissimus dorsi, triceps, forearm and hand flexors |

PROBLEM AREAS:

Knee
Wrist
Muscular fatigue

AREAS TO EMPHASIZE:

- Knee—strengthen the knee joint to meet the increased demands on the knee.

- Arms and shoulders—develop the musculature involved with delivering the ball in order to minimize muscular fatigue.

---

*The editor is grateful to Major Pat Simpson for his assistance in writing this chapter.

## Table 16-2. Bowling Nautilus Workout Program

| EXERCISE<br>(in order) | PRIMARY MUSCLES<br>DEVELOPED | SPECIFIC SKILLS<br>INVOLVED |
|---|---|---|
| 1. Leg Extension | Quadriceps | Approach, strengthen knee joint |
| 2. Leg Curl | Hamstrings | Approach; strengthen knee joint |
| 3. Double Shoulder (lateral raise) | Deltoids | Backswing with the ball; delivery |
| 4. Double Shoulder (seated press) | Deltoids, triceps | Backswing and delivery |
| 5. Pullover | Latissimus dorsi | Backswing and delivery |
| 6. Biceps Curl | Biceps | Release of the ball |
| 7. Wrist Curl | Forearm flexors | Grip and release of the ball |
| 8. Squeeze a rubber ball | Forearm and hand flexors | Grip |

- Perform 1 set of 8 to 12 reps of each exercise

- Take no more than 60 seconds to perform each set

- Rest no more than 30 seconds between each set

- To determine **total workout time**: multiply # of workouts by 1½ minutes, then subtract 30 seconds from total

## Table 16-3. Bowling Universal Workout Program

| | EXERCISE (in order) | PRIMARY MUSCLES DEVELOPED | SPECIFIC SKILLS INVOLVED |
|---|---|---|---|
| 1. | Leg Extension | Quadriceps | Approach |
| 2. | Leg Curl | Hamstrings | Approach |
| 3. | Bench Press | Pectorals, deltoids, triceps | Delivery of the ball |
| 4. | Lat Pulldown | Latissimus dorsi, biceps | Backswing with the ball |
| 5. | Seated Press | Delfoids, triceps | Backswing and delivery |
| 6. | Upright Rowing | Deltoids, biceps | Backswing and delivery |
| 7. | Wrist Curls | Forearm flexors | Grip and release of the ball |
| 8. | Squeezing a rubber ball | Forearm and hand flexors | Grip |

- Perform 1 set of 8 to 12 reps of each exercise
- Take no more than 60 seconds to perform each set
- Rest no more than 30 seconds between each set
- To determine **total workout time**: multiply # of workouts by 1½ minutes, then subtract 30 seconds from total

# CHAPTER 17
## Boxing

Boxing is an activity which requires extraordinately high levels of stamina, muscular endurance, and explosive power. All of these requirements can be developed by means of a properly-planned conditioning program. Such a program should improve several aspects of boxing: the ability of the boxer to keep holding his hands at the proper level; the ability of the athlete to be hit without resulting in either undue discomfort or a serious injury; the ability of the individual to forcefully throw punches; the ability of the boxer to *sustain* a minimum level of forceful punching; and the ability of the participant to move quickly, gracefully, and purposefully while boxing.

There are several drills which can effectively augment a conditioning program for boxing. Included in such drills are: the squared-up power punching drill; jumping rope; spring-jog drills; and boxing practice rounds (both shadow and actual boxing).

In the squared-up, power punching drill, the athlete stands with his feet squared-up to the hanging punching bag approximately one straight arm's length distance away. Starting with both hands on his chin, the boxer alternates his hands and strikes the bag with a straight punch (palms down) as forcefully as he can. This drill is designed to develop endurance in the musculature involved with throwing punches. As a general rule, boxers should regularly jump rope (recommended time — 15-20 minutes daily 4-5 times a week). In sprint-jog drills, the athlete performs a continuous series of short (15-20 years) runs, alternating vigorous sprints with recovery bouts of jogging. The recommended dosage is approximately five minutes. Practice rounds provide not only exercise, but also increased neuromuscular efficiency.

## Table 16-1. Boxing overview

| BASIC SKILLS | MUSCLES INVOLVED |
|---|---|
| 1. Punching | Latissimus dorsi, deltoids, triceps, biceps, pectorals, buttocks, trunk flexors |
| 2. Footwork | Buttocks, quadriceps, hamstrings gastrocnemius |

PROBLEM AREAS:

Neck
Abdominals
Wrists
Stamina
Muscular fatigue

AREAS TO EMPHASIZE:

- Neck—develop all movements of the neck to prevent serious injury

- Abdominals—strengthen abdominals to enable athlete to better sustain a punch to the stomach

- Arms and shoulders—develop the musculature used in throwing a punch in order to delay the onslaught of fatigue produced by throwing punches

## Table 17-2. Off-season Boxing Nautilus Workout Program

| EXERCISE (in order) | PRIMARY MUSCLES DEVELOPED | SPECIFIC SKILLS INVOLVED |
|---|---|---|
| 1. Leg Extension* | Quadriceps | Footwork, movement |
| 2. Leg Press* | Buttocks, quadriceps | Footwork, movement |
| 3. Leg Curl* | Hamstrings | Footwork, movement |
| 4. Double Chest* (bent arm fly) | Pectorals | Punching |
| 5. Double Chest (decline press) | Pectorals, deltoids, triceps | Punching, holding up gloves |
| 6. Chin-ups* | Latissimus dorsi, biceps | Punching |
| 7. Double Shoulder* (lateral raise) | Deltoids | Punching, holding up gloves |
| 8. Double Shoulder* (seated press) | Deltoids, triceps | Punching, holding up gloves |
| 9. Shrugs* | Trapezius | Stabilize shoulder girdle, holding up gloves |
| 10. Wrist Curl* | Forearm flexors | Wrist support |
| 11. Situps* | Abdominals | Stabilize abdominal wall |
| 12. 4-Way Neck* | Neck flexors and extensors | Stabilize head and neck; reduce injury possibility |

- Perform 1 set of 8 to 12 reps of each exercise
- Take no more than 60 seconds to perform each set
- Rest no more than 30 seconds between each set
- To determine **total workout time**: multiply # of workouts by 1½ minutes, then subtract 30 seconds from total

*In-season only

## Table 17-3. Off-season Boxing Universal Workout Program

| EXERCISE (in order) | PRIMARY MUSCLES DEVELOPED | SPECIFIC SKILLS INVOLVED |
|---|---|---|
| 1. Leg Press* | Buttocks, quadriceps | Footwork, movement |
| 2. Leg Extension* | Quadriceps | Footwork, movement |
| 3. Leg Curl* | Hamstrings | Footwork, movement |
| 4. Bench Press* | Pectorals, deltoids, triceps | Punching; holding up the gloves |
| 5. Lat Pulldown* | Latissimus dorsi, biceps | Punching |
| 6. Seated Press* | Deltoids, triceps | Punching, holding up the gloves |
| 7. Upright Rowing | Deltoids, triceps | Punching, prevent elbow hyperextension |
| 8. Triceps Extension* | Triceps | Punching |
| 9. Wrist Curl* | Forearm flexors | Support the wrists |
| 10. Situps* | Abdominals | Stabilize the abdominal wall |
| 11. Neck Station* | Neck flexors & extensors | Stabilize the neck; reduce the possibility of injury |
| 12. Shrugs* | Trapezius | Holding up the glove |

- Perform 1 set of 8 to 12 reps of each exercise
- Take no more than 60 seconds to perform each set
- Rest no more than 30 seconds between each set
- To determine **total workout time**: multiply # of workouts by 1½ minutes, then subtract 30 seconds from total

*In-season only

# CHAPTER 18
## Field Hockey

Field hockey is one of the most strenuous, physically demanding activities played by women. Every field hockey player must possess a high level of physical fitness for maximum performance. All of the basic components of fitness (muscular strength, muscular endurance, flexibility, and cardiovascular fitness) are required to play competitive field hockey.

Since field hockey involves continuous running, an adequate level of stamina is a MUST! In general, developing stamina for field hockey is best accomplished by fartlek training (alternating sprints and jogging) rather than prolonged bouts of merely jogging. Jogging laps around the hockey field simply does not adequately prepare the athlete for the 'Stop and Go' nature of the game. Ten to fifteen minutes of wind sprints of 25, 50 and 75 yards with quick stops and turns should be included in all practices. In addition, the athlete should be required to run while working on stickwork—such as dribbling, receiving and passing. There are also several exercises which can contribute to improving the stamina requirements for the game: running-in-place, jumping-in-place (and in different directions—e.g. forward, back, right and left); jumping jacks; and rope jumping.

Flexibility exercises should also be an integral part of the daily workout. Warm-ups which stretch specific muscle groups are essential to relatively injury-free and efficient play. The daily warm-up period should include lower back, leg and shoulder girdle flexibility exercises. The following exercises performed slowly and smoothly can be included in the program: sitting toe touches (with legs together and apart); hurdle position toe touches; standing toe touches (with legs together and apart); arm circles; and arm flings.

In addition to the aforementioned program factors, athletes interested in improving their performance level in field hockey should also engage in a regular program of muscular development. Such a program should be augmented with efforts to develop the appropriate motor abilities utilized in field hockey and a preventive-injury program (especially the athlete's feet).

*The editor is grateful to Susan L. Peterson for her assistance in writing this chapter.

Table 18-1. Field hockey overview

| BASIC SKILLS | MUSCLES INVOLVED |
|---|---|
| 1. Running | Quadriceps, hamstrings, buttocks |
| 2. Passing  stickwork 3. Receiving | Latissimus dorsi, deltoids, triceps, pectorals, biceps |
| 4. Shooting | Latissimus dorsi, pectorals, deltoids, triceps |

PROBLEM AREAS:

Stamina
Grip strength
Muscular fatigue
Knee injuries

AREAS TO EMPHASIZE:

- Grip—develop both the forearm and the hand flexors

- Arms and shoulder—develop the musculature involved with both shooting the ball and stick handling in order to decrease the severity of muscular fatigue.

- Knee—develop the musculature of the leg so that violent collisions will not result in knee injuries

## Table 18-2. Off-season Field Hockey Nautilus Workout Program

| EXERCISE (in order) | PRIMARY MUSCLES DEVELOPED | SPECIFIC SKILLS INVOLVED |
|---|---|---|
| 1. Leg Extension* | Quadriceps | Running |
| 2. Leg Press | Buttocks, quadriceps | Running |
| 3. Hip and Back* | Buttocks, lower back | Running |
| 4. Leg Curl* | Hamstrings | Runnings |
| 5. Double Shoulder* (lateral raise) | Deltoids | Shooting, stickwork |
| 6. Double Shoulder (seated press) | Deltoids, triceps | Shooting, stickwork |
| 7. Shrugs* | Trapezius | Stickwork |
| 8. Pullover | Latissimus dorsi | Shooting, stickwork |
| 9. Chins* | Latissimus dorsi, biceps | Stickwork |
| 10. Dips* | Pectorals, deltoids, triceps | Shooting, stickwork |
| 11. Biceps Curl | Biceps | Stickwork |
| 12. Wrist Curls* | Forearm flexors | Grip, dribble |

- Perform 1 set of 8 to 12 reps of each exercise during off-season
- Take no more than 60 seconds to perform each set
- Rest no more than 30 seconds between each set
- To determine **total workout time**: multiply # of workouts by 1½ minutes, then subtract 30 seconds from total

*In-season only

## Table 18-3. Off-season Field Hockey Universal Workout Program

| EXERCISE (in order) | PRIMARY MUSCLES DEVELOPED | SPECIFIC SKILLS INVOLVED |
|---|---|---|
| 1. Leg Press* | Buttocks, quadriceps | Running |
| 2. Leg Extension* | Quadriceps | Running |
| 3. Leg Curl* | Hamstrings | Running |
| 4. Bench Press* | Pectorals, deltoids, triceps | Shooting, stickwork |
| 5. Lat Pulldown* | Latissimus dorsi, biceps | Stickwork |
| 6. Seated Press* | Deltoids, triceps | Shooting, stickwork |
| 7. Upright Row* | Deltoids, Biceps | Shooting, stickwork |
| 8. Triceps Extension | Triceps | Shooting, stickwork |
| 9. Biceps Curl | Biceps | Stickwork |
| 10. Wrist Curls* | Forearm flexors | Grip, dribbling |
| 11. Squeezing a rubber ball | Forearm and hand flexors | Grip, dribbling |

- Perform 1 set of 8 to 12 reps of each exercise during off-season
- Take no more than 60 seconds to perform each set
- Rest no more than 30 seconds between each set
- To determine **total workout time:** multiply # of workouts by 1½ minutes, then subtract 30 seconds from total

*In-season only

# CHAPTER 19
## Football

As one of the nation's most popular participant and spectator sports, football is played and watched by millions of individuals across the country every weekend during the season. The action on the gridiron is affected by a number of factors: the strategy employed by the opposing coaches; the inherent abilities of the two teams; and the collective dedication to *winning* exhibited by the individual players. One commonality which affects all three of the aforementioned factors is the physical fitness level of the team members. A coach whose team is faster and stronger than his opponent will develop a strategy to take advantage of his team's assets. A player who possesses a high level of personal fitness is better equipped to perform on the football field.

Individuals who are physically fit can translate their emotional commitment to winning into tangible performances on the gridiron. Without question, the primary fitness component for the football player is muscular fitness.

Muscular strength is the basis for every powerful, explosive movement made by a football player during a game. Muscular fitness also helps protect an athlete against the possibility of injuries. Not only do stronger muscles enable the football player to block and tackle better, run faster, and kick and run farther; but they also provide increased joint stability, thus protecting the vulnerable neck, shoulder, elbow, wrist, hip, knee, and ankle joints. In addition, muscular strength improves the performance of a football player by increasing the endurance level of the many muscles utilized during a game. A high degree of muscular endurance enables a football player to minimize the muscular fatigue which so frequently limits athletic performance.

To some degree, a majority of all football players and coaches recognize the role that muscular strength plays in developing a successful team. As a result, most teams engage in a strength-training program of some sort. A large number of these programs, however, do not achieve the maximum level of results possible; especially when the time and effort put into these programs by everyone involved is considered. Faulty training techniques and a lack of understanding of the basic principles of exercise are the typical reasons for such a shortcoming.

Although virtually all of an individual's muscles are used when playing football, weight training programs for the football players should concentrate on developing strong shoulders, arms, the lower back, and

*The editor is grateful to Major Alfred Rushatz for his assistance in writing this chapter.

upper legs. Likewise, the muscular development program for a football player should strengthen the neck, increase joint stability, and increase and maintain the joint flexibility required to prevent serious injuries.

Table 19-1. Football overview

| BASIC SKILLS | MUSCLES INVOLVED |
|---|---|
| 1. Passing a football | Forearm flexors, triceps, deltoids, trapezius |
| 2. Tackling | Pectorals, deltoids, triceps, trunk flexors |
| 3. Blocking | Lower back muscles, hamstrings, buttocks |
| 4. Running | Quadriceps, hamstrings, buttocks |
| 5. Kicking | Quadriceps, illiopsoas |
| 6. Hand shivers | Triceps |

PROBLEM AREAS:

Stamina
Muscular fatigue
Neck injuries
Knee injuries
Shoulder injuries

AREAS TO EMPHASIZE:

- Develop stamina by means of a comprehensive running/interval program

- Develop the musculature involved in the basic skills of footballs.

- Emphasize extensive flexibility conditioning

- Develop the musculature of the neck

- Develop the knee joint

## Table 19-2. Off-season Football Nautilus Workout Program

| EXERCISE (in order) | PRIMARY MUSCLES DEVELOPED | SPECIFIC SKILLS INVOLVED |
|---|---|---|
| 1. Hip and Back* | Buttocks, lower back | Running, tackling, blocking |
| 2. Leg Extension* | Quadriceps | Running, tackling, kicking |
| 3. Leg Press | Buttocks, quadriceps | Running, tackling, blocking, kicking |
| 4. Leg Curl* | Hamstrings | Running forward, sidward, and backward |
| 5. Double Shoulder* (lateral raise) | Deltoids | Tackling, blocking, throwing |
| 6. Double Shoulder* (seated press) | Deltoids, triceps | Tackling, blocking, throwing |
| 7. Pullover* | Latissimus dorsi, biceps | Blocking, tackling, blocking |
| 8. Chins* | Latissimus dorsi, biceps | Blocking, tackling, throwing |
| 9. Dips | Pectorals, deltoids, triceps | Tackling, blocking, throwing |
| 10. Biceps Curls | Biceps | Tackling, blocking, throwing |
| 11. Triceps Extension | Triceps | Throwing, hitting, tackling |
| 12. Four-Way Neck | *Neck muscles | Protect neck during tackling, blocking |
| 13. Shrugs* | Trapezius | Protect against neck injuries and AC separations |

- Perform 1 set of 8 to 12 reps of each exercise during off-season
- Take no more than 60 seconds to perform each set
- Rest no more than 30 seconds between each set
- To determine **total workout time:** multiply # of workouts by 1½ minutes, then subtract 30 seconds from total

*In-season only

## Table 19-3. Off-season Football Universal Workout Program

| EXERCISE (in order) | PRIMARY MUSCLES DEVELOPED | SPECIFIC SKILLS INVOLVED |
|---|---|---|
| 1. Leg Press* | Buttocks, quadriceps | Running, blocking, tackling |
| 2. Leg Raises* | Quadriceps | Running, tackling, kicking, blocking |
| 3. Leg Curl* | Hamstrings | Running forward, sideward and backward |
| 4. Bench Press* | Pectorals, deltoids, triceps | Tackling, blocking, throwing |
| 5. Chin-ups* | Latissimus dorsi, biceps | Throwing, tackling, blocking |
| 6. Seated press* | Deltoids, triceps | Tackling, blocking, throwing |
| 7. Upright rowing* | Deltoids, biceps, trapezius | Tackling, blocking |
| 8. Hyper extension* | Lower back | Tackling, blocking |
| 9. Triceps extension | Triceps | Blocking, tackling, throwing |
| 10. Biceps Curl | Biceps | Tackling, hitting, throwing |
| 11. Neck Station* | Neck muscles | Protect neck from injury |
| 12. Shrugs* | Trapezius | Protect neck from injury |

- Perform 1 set of 8 to 12 reps of each exercise during off-season
- Take no more than 60 seconds to perform each set
- Rest no more than 30 seconds between each set
- To determine **total workout time:** multiply # of workouts by 1½ minutes, then subtract 30 seconds from total

*In-season only

## Table 19-4. Off-season Football Stretching, Flexibility, Speed and Endurance Program

A. Stretching and Flexibility:
The purpose of stretching is to prevent injuries and prepare the muscles for activity.
1. Individual Stretching:
   a. Standing
      (1) Wing stretch—Touch hands together in the back. Do 5 reps., 5 times.
      (2) Ankle rollers—Walk on the outsides and then the insides for 5 yards.
      (3) Figure 8—Run a figure 8 around the goal post or around an imaginary point.
      (4) Standing leg straddle—Spread the leg, knees straight and bring the head to the knee. Hold for 5 count and do to other legs.
   b. Sitting
      (1) Spread legs—Touch the toes while having the legs and back straight. Hold for count of 5.
      (2) Hurdlers stretch—Touch toes while keeping the legs and back straight. Then alternate legs.
      (3) Both legs together—Both hands try and touch toes to a count of 5.
   c. Lying on the stomach—Grasp left ankle with right hand and pull. Hold for 5 count and reverse.
   d. Lying on the back—
      (1) Alternate toe touch—Touch toe to hand, hold to a count of 5 and then reverse.
      (2) Sitting on ankles—Bend backwards while sitting on the ankles and touch the head or back to the ground.
      (3) Knees to chest—Alternate legs to chest. Use hands to pull the leg the last part and hold to a 5 count. Bring both legs to the chest at the same time and hold for 5.
2. Partner stretch:
   a. On the back—
      (1) Groin stretch—Slightly spread legs with your partner standing inside the knees of the down person. The down person presses against the partners legs to a count of 5. Change and partners feet outside the knees and have the down person spread his legs to a count of 5.
   2. Leg lifts—Partner puts his fingers on the down persons toes and the down man lifts to a 5 count against mild pressure.
   b. On the stomach
      Hamstring stretch — The down has his legs bent at a 90° angle. Parnter holds ankles and the down man pulls 5 times to a count of 5. Next, the down man pushes against his partne's hands. The same count and number of repetitions applies.
3. STRETCHING SHOULD BE PERFORMED AT LEAST 3-4 TIMES A WEEK
B. Speed and Endurance:
1. Endurance—
   a. Jog 325 yards around a football field with a minutes rest between laps. Do this 2 times rest for 5 minutes and then repeat. Each week increase 1 lap, until 6 laps have been reached.
   b. Continually check the heart beat in order to keep it between 150 and 160 beats per minute.
   c. Run 3 minutes of steps without stopping 3 times per week.
2. Speed—
   a. Sprint 30 yards 10 times with 15 seconds rest between each sprint. Rest 2 2 minutes and then repeat once.
   b. Increase 5 sprints every 2 weeks.
3. The endurance and speed workouts should be performed on days when the athlete does not weight train.

# CHAPTER 20
## Golf

Golf is an activity demanding a very high degree of refined motor skills. As in any other activity, nothing can replace the practice and repetition of the specific skills associated with playing the game.

Most golfers would not make a significant connection between their level of strength and success in competition because golf is not generally regarded as a strength-related activity. In fact, few players, aside from the professionals, ever undertake a program of physical exercise specifically designed to enhance their performance; most of us consider the activity itself an adequate form of preparation. Nothing could be further from the truth.

Ben Hogan is widely recognized as a master teacher of the game. In addition to being a champion player, Hogan has devoted a lifetime of study to the physiology of what he terms the "repeating swing." The repeating swing is one which the player can execute with surety despite mental and physical fatigue, and under great tension in the face of competitive pressure. Because the golf swing is nothing more than a series of muscle movements, although admittedly refined ones, it stands to reason that some attention should be given the muscles themselves. An increase in strength can improve a golfer's performance by increasing the endurance of the muscles involved. This increase in strength will prevent or delay the onset of fatigue of those muscles instrumental in executing the repeating swing. It will also aid in maintaining the player's confidence, an important ingredient in handling tension, avoiding mental fatigue.

Strength in itself will not enable the individual to hit the ball better or longer. However, it will allow the skilled player to strike shots with more consistent explosive power over more extended periods. In other words, for the **skilled** player, strength **does** translate directly into greater distance and improved endurance.

The muscles specific to the golfer are those of the hips and legs, the shoulder girdle, the forearms and hands (grip strength).

*The editor is grateful to Major Paul Kirkegaard, head golf coach at USMA, for his assistance in writing this chapter.

Table 20-1. Golf overview

| BASIC SKILLS | MUSCLES INVOLVED |
|---|---|
| 1. Driving power | Buttocks, quadriceps, hamstrings, lower back muscles |
| 2. Hip turn | Lower back muscles, hip flexors |
| 3. Impact velocity | Latissimus dorsi, triceps |
| 4. Club extension | Deltoids, triceps |
| 5. Clubhead control | Triceps, biceps, forearm and hand flexors |
| 6. Walking endurance | Buttocks, quadriceps |

PROBLEM AREAS:

Muscular fatigue
Hand injuries (blisters, etc.)
Walking stamina
Joint aches and discomfort

AREAS TO EMPHASIZE:

- Develop the forearm and hand flexors to protect hand and wrist injuries

- Develop the musculature used in the golf swing to delay or prevent muscular fatigue.

- Warm-up properly

- Perform flexibility exercises on a regular basis

# Golf

## Table 20-2. A Nautilus Workout Program for Golf*

| EXERCISE (in order) | PRIMARY MUSCLES DEVELOPED | SPECIFIC SKILLS INVOLVED |
|---|---|---|
| 1. Hip and Back | Buttocks, lower back | Driving power, walking endurance |
| 2. Leg Extension | Quadriceps | Driving power, walking endurance |
| 3. Leg Curl | Hamstrings | Hip turn and driving power |
| 4. Double Shoulder (lateral raise) | Deltoids | Club Control, impact velocity |
| 5. Double Shoulder (seated press) | Deltoids, triceps | Shoulder turn, club extension |
| 6. Pull Over | Latissimus Dorsi | Shoulder turn, club extension |
| 7. Wrist Curl | Forearm flexors | Clubhead control, impact power, acceleration |
| 8. Reverse Wrist Curls | Forearm flexors | Clubhead control, impact power, acceleration |

*Golf is generally a year-around activity.
- Perform 1 set of 8 to 12 reps of each exercise.
- Take no more than 60 seconds to perform each set
- Rest no more than 30 seconds between each set
- To determine *total workout time*: multiply # of workouts by 1½ minutes, then subtract 30 seconds from total.

## Table 20-3. A Universal Workout Program for Golf*

| EXERCISE (in order) | PRIMARY MUSCLES DEVELOPED | SPECIFIC SKILLS INVOLVED |
|---|---|---|
| 1. Leg Press | Buttocks, quadriceps | Driving power, walking endurance |
| 2. Leg Extension | Quadriceps | Driving power, walking endurance |
| 3. Leg Curl | Hamstrings | Hip turn, driving power |
| 4. Lat Pulldown | Latissimus dorsi, biceps | Club control, impact velocity |
| 5. Seated Press | Deltoids, triceps | Shoulder turn, club extension |
| 6. Upright Rowing | Deltoids, biceps | Shoulder turn, club extension |
| 7. Wrist Curls | Forearm flexors | Clubhead control, impact power, acceleration |
| 8. Reverse Wrist Curls | Forearm extensors | Clubhead control, impact power, acceleration |

*Golf is generally a year-around activity

- Perform 1 set of 8 to 12 reps of each exercise
- Take no more than 60 seconds to perform each set
- Rest no more than 30 seconds between each set
- To determine *total workout time*: multiply # of workouts by 1½ minutes, then subtract 30 seconds from total.

# CHAPTER 21
## Gymnastics

Success in gymnastics cannot be achieved, to any great extent, without the athlete possessing fundamental physical skills and abilities. At the heart of these abilities is a high level of physical fitness. As such, improvement in the skills involved in gymnastics is best achieved by **both** practice of the skills and a properly-planned program of conditioning performed on a regular basis—both in and out-of-season.

Since gymnastics is a sport which involves numerous gross and fine motor skills utilizing **all** of the major muscles of the body, the gymnast should undertake an overall muscular development program. Within limits, an improvement in an athlete's level of muscular fitness can result not only in consistently better performance in the individual's existing gymnastics routine, but also in the development of new skills, new routines, and new avenues of skill exploration. Regardless of the program adopted for muscular fitness improvement, the conditioning regimen **must** include an extensive program of flexibility exercises (refer to Chapter 13 for specific exercises).

*The editor is grateful to Larry Butler, assistant gymnastics coach at USMA, for his assistance in writing this chapter.

## Table 21-1. Gymnastics overview

| BASIC SKILLS | MUSCLES INVOLVED |
|---|---|
| 1. Vaulting | Buttocks, lower back, quadriceps |
| 2. Pressing movement (e.g. P-bars) | Deltoids, triceps, pectorals |
| 3. Pulling movement | Latissimus dorsi, biceps |
| 4. Straight arm lever (e.g. hand balance) | Pectorals, deltoids |
| 5. Trampoline and tumbling | Illiopsoas, sartorius |
| 6. Floor exercise | Buttocks, lower back, quadriceps, deltoids, triceps, pectorals |

PROBLEM AREAS:

Muscular fatigue
Muscular soreness
Flexibility
Ankle injuries

AREAS TO EMPHASIZE:

- Develop the musculature involved in the specific gymnastics skills to prevent muscular fatigue

- Develop joint (ankle, knee, shoulder) stability to minimize the possibility of injuries

- Include flexibility exercises in the workout on a regular basis.

- Warm-up thoroughly

## Table 21-2. Off-season Gymnastics Nautilus Workout Program

| EXERCISE (in order) | PRIMARY MUSCLES DEVELOPED | SPECIFIC SKILLS INVOLVED |
|---|---|---|
| 1. Hip and Back* | Buttocks, lower back | Running, jumping, vaulting, floor exercise |
| 2. Leg Extension* | Quadriceps | Vaulting, floor exercise, jumping |
| 3. Leg Press | Buttocks, Quadriceps | Vaulting, floor exercises, jumping, trampoline |
| 4. Leg Curl* | Hamstrings | Running |
| 5. Double Shoulder* (lateral raise) | Deltoids | Pressing movements on P. bars, rings, pommel, horse, floor exercise, supports |
| 6. Double Shoulder* (seated press) | Deltoids, triceps | Pressing movements on apparatus and floor exercise supports |
| 7. Shrug | Trapezius | Extension and stabilization of the shoulder girdle |
| 8. Pullover* | Latissimus Dorsi | Pulling movements on the apparatus |
| 10. Dips | Pectorals, deltoids, triceps | Pressing movements on apparatus and floor exercise |
| 11. Biceps Curls | Biceps | Pulling movements on the apparatus |
| 12. Wrist Curls* | Forearm flexors | Grip strength on all apparatus |

- Perform 1 set of 8 to 12 reps of each exercise
- Take no more than 60 seconds to perform each set
- Rest no more than 30 seconds between each set
- To determine *total workout time*: multiply # of workouts by 1½ minutes, then subtract 30 seconds from total

*In-season only; some high-level gymnasts are in-season the year around. These athletes should lift twice a week, schedule permitting.

## Table 21-3. Off-season Gymnastics Universal Workout Program

| EXERCISE (in order) | PRIMARY MUSCLES DEVELOPED | SPECIFIC SKILLS INVOLVED |
|---|---|---|
| 1. Leg Press* | Buttocks, quadriceps | Running, jumping, vaulting, tumbling, trampoline |
| 2. Leg Extension | Quadriceps | Running, jumping, vaulting, tumbling |
| 3. Leg Curl* | Hamstrings | Running |
| 4. Bench Press* | Pectorals, deltoids, triceps | Supports, extensions, balances, straight arm lever |
| 5. Chin-ups* | Latissimus dorsi, biceps | Pulling movements |
| 6. Seated Press* | Deltoids, triceps | Supports, hand balancing |
| 7. Upright Rowing* | Deltoids, biceps | Supports, hand balancing |
| 8. Hyperextension | Trapezius | Elevating and depressing the shoulder girdle |
| 9. Shrugs | Lower back | Tumbling, pike opening, front somersault |
| 10. Triceps Extension | Triceps | Supports, extensions, balances on apparatus and floor |
| 11. Biceps Curl | Biceps | Pulling movements on apparatus |
| 12. Wrist Curl* | Forearm flexors | Grip strength on all apparatus |

- Perform 1 set of 8 to 12 reps of each exercise
- Take no more than 60 seconds to perform each set
- Rest no more than 30 seconds between each set
- To determine *total workout time:* multiply # of workouts by 1½ minutes, then subtract 30 seconds from total

*In season only; some high-level gymnasts are in-season the year around. These athletes should lift twice a week, schedule permitting.

Table 21-4. Conditioning exercises for gymnasts.

---

**1. Handstand Push-ups** — Handstand push-ups should be performed on low parallel bars, using a partner. The gymnast kicks up to a handstand and the partner grabs his legs. The gymnast bends his arms and lowers down to a shoulder stand and then pushes back up to the handstand. He performs as many repetitions as possible and when he can no longer do them by himself the spotter helps to lift and balance him.

**2. Front level pull-ups** — Hang on the high bar or rings and lift one knee so the thigh is perpendicular to the floor. Pull the body up so that it becomes parallel to the floor (front lever position). Hold this position for several seconds then do a pull up. At the top of the pull-up begin to lower back down to the front lever position and hold it for several seconds. Repeat this sequence as many times as possible.

**3. Dips on parallel bars** — Support the body with straight arms on the parallel bars and have a partner grab the gymnast's ankles. Bend the arms and lower the body down slowly. Have the partner pull down on the ankles. Then push back up and have the partner offer resistance. The partner should offer sufficient resistance so that the gymnast can only perform between 8-12 repetitions.

**4. Leg raises and form drill** — The gymnast begins by lying on his back on a mat and grabbing onto the ankles of a partner who is standing over him. With straight knees and pointed toes, the gymnast should attempt to kick the partner with his feet. The partner catches his feet and pushes them down to the floor vigorously. The gymnast should not let his feet hit the floor. He should immediately attempt to kick the partner again. This exercise is performed for 30 seconds.

**5. Handstand walk** — This is a very simple, but effective exercise. The gymnast simply walks on his hands across the length of the floor exercise mat. He should attempt to walk back and forth as many times as possible. If necessary, a partner can help balance him so that he can continue.

---

# CHAPTER 22
## Handball

Handball is a sport which requires substantial levels of **every** major component of physical fitness. Stamina is essential because even for the individual who only plays handball on an occasional basis, the game involves extensive running. On the average, more than half the time spent in the court by two players of approximately equal ability is spent running. An adequate level of muscular development is important, not only to provide an appropriate level of power for stroking the ball, but also to permit the handball player to maintain the precision and muscular endurance essential to successful handball. In addition, adequate flexibility is a basic requirement for "winning handball." Although all of the information presented in Part I of this test can be of benefit to the handball player (at any level), **particular** attention should be paid to the sections on interval training, injury prevention, flexibility and muscular development. Depending on the time available and the level of fitness of the player, conditioning for handball should be undertaken a minimum of 2-3 times per week.

Table 22-1. Handball overview

| BASIC SKILLS | MUSCLES INVOLVED |
|---|---|
| 1. Hitting the ball | Latissimus dorsi, triceps, deltoids |
| 2. Putting "hop" on the ball | Forearm flexors; biceps |
| 3. Running | Quadriceps, hamstrings, buttocks |
| 4. Changing directions while moving | Buttocks, calf muscles, quadriceps |

PROBLEM AREAS:

Elbow injuries
Knee injuries
Stamina
Muscular endurance
Shoulder injuries

AREAS TO EMPHASIZE:

- Proper warm-up

- Develop elbow, knee, and shoulder joints to prevent injuries

- Develop the musculature involved in handball to minimize muscular fatigue

- Utilize interval training to develop stamina

- Emphasize flexibility conditioning exercises

Table 22-2. Handball Nautilus Workout Program*

| EXERCISE (in order) | PRIMARY MUSCLES DEVELOPED | SPECIFIC SKILLS INVOLVED |
|---|---|---|
| 1. Leg Extension | Quadriceps | Running |
| 2. Leg Press | Buttocks, Quadriceps | Running |
| 3. Hip and Back | Buttocks | Running |
| 4. Leg Curl | Hamstrings | Running |
| 5. Double-shoulder (lateral raise) | Deltoids | Stroking the ball, prevent shoulder injuries |
| 6. Double-shoulder (seated press) | Deltoids, triceps | Stroking the ball, prevent shoulder injuries |
| 7. Pullover | Latissimus dorsi | Stroking the ball |
| 8. Biceps Curl | Biceps | Prevent elbow injuries, rotating the hand while hitting the ball |
| 9. Triceps Extension | Triceps | Hitting the ball |
| 10. Wrist Curl | Forearm flexors | Hitting the ball, putting 'hop' on the ball |

*Handball is generally a year-around sport
• Perform 1 set of 8 to 12 reps of each exercise
• Take no more than 60 seconds to perform each set
• Rest no more than 30 seconds between each set
• To determine *total workout time:* multiply # of workouts by 1½ minutes, then subtract 30 second from total.

## Table 22-3. Handball Universal Workout Program*

| EXERCISE (in order) | PRIMARY MUSCLES DEVELOPED | SPECIFIC SKILLS INVOLVED |
|---|---|---|
| 1. Leg Press | Buttocks, quadriceps | Running |
| 2. Leg Extension | Quadriceps | Running |
| 3. Leg Curl | Hamstrings | Running |
| 4. Seated Press | Deltoids, triceps | Hitting the ball, prevent shoulder injury |
| 5. Lat Pulldown | Latissimus dorsi, biceps | Hitting the ball |
| 6. Bench Press (or dip) | Pectorals, deltoids, Triceps | Hitting the ball |
| 7. Upright Row | Deltoids, biceps | Hitting the ball, prevent shoulder injuries |
| 8. Triceps Extension | Triceps | Hitting the ball, prevent prevent elbow injuries |
| 9. Biceps Curl | Biceps | Prevent elbow injuries; rotating the hand while hitting the ball |
| 10. Wrist Curl | Forearm flexors | Hitting one ball, put 'hop' on the ball |

*Handball is generally a year-around sport

- Perform 1 set of 8 to 12 reps of each exercise
- Take no more than 60 seconds to perform each set
- Rest no more than 30 seconds between each set
- To determine *total workout time:* multiply # of workouts by 1½ minutes, then subtract 30 seconds from total.

# CHAPTER 23
## Ice Hockey

Often referred to as "the fastest sport" in the world, ice hockey is a rigorous, physically-demanding activity. To be a successful hockey player, an athlete must possess a high level of muscular fitness, cardiovascular fitness, flexibility, and motor abilities. In short, ice hockey requires **total conditioning.** Leg strength enables the skater to move faster. Strength in the shoulders, arms, wrists, and lower back provides the basis for quick, explosive shooting of the puck. Muscular endurance permits the ice hockey player to sustain his level of performance while on the ice. And finally, an adequate level of cardiovascular fitness ensures that the athlete will have sufficient aerobic stamina to meet the substantial demands placed on his heart and lungs by this fast-moving game.

The core of the conditioning program for ice hockey should concentrate on muscular fitness improvement. Such a program should be augmented with regular bouts of flexibility exercising and interval training.

*The editor is grateful to James W. Zuckermandel for his assistance in writing this chapter.

Table 23-1. Ice hockey overview

| BASIC SKILLS | MUSCLES INVOLVED |
|---|---|
| 1. Skating | Buttocks, quadriceps, hamstrings |
| 2. Shooting | Pectorals, deltoids, triceps, biceps, latissimus dorsi, forearm flexors |
| 3. Checking | *all* major muscles |

PROBLEM AREAS:

Stamina
Muscular fatigue
Knee injuries
Shoulder injuries

AREAS TO EMPHASIZE:

- Develop forearm and hand flexors for improved gripping ability
- Develop stamina by a regular program of cardiovascular conditioning (e.g. circuit training, interval training, running, skating)
- Develop joint stability (knee and shoulder particularly) to minimize the possibility of injuries
- Develop the musculature involved in ice hockey to prevent musculature fatigue
- Include flexibility exercises in the workout program
- Warm-up properly

## Table 23-2. Off-season Ice Hockey Nautilus Workout Program

| EXERCISE (in order) | PRIMARY MUSCLES DEVELOPED | SPECIFIC SKILLS INVOLVED |
|---|---|---|
| 1. Hip and Back* | Buttocks, quadriceps | Skating, shooting |
| 2. Leg Extension* | Quadriceps | Skating |
| 3. Leg Press | Buttocks, quadriceps | Skating |
| 4. Leg Curl* | Hamstrings | Skating |
| 5. Double Shoulder (lateral raise) | Deltoids | Shooting, checking |
| 6. Double Shoulder (seated press) | Deltoids, triceps | Shooting |
| 7. Shrug | Trapezius | Shooting |
| 8. Pullover | Latissimus dorsi | Shooting |
| 9. Chins* | Latissimus dorsi, biceps | Shooting, checking |
| 10. Dips* | Pectorals, deltoids, triceps | Shooting, checking |
| 11. Wrist Curls* | Forearm flexors | Shooting, wrist strength, and control |
| 12. Reverse Curls | Forearm extensors | Shooting, wrist strength and control |

*In-season only

- Perform 1 set of 8 to 12 reps of each exercise
- Take no more than 60 seconds to perform each set
- Rest no more than 30 seconds between each set
- To determine *total workout time:* multiply # of workouts by 1½ minutes, then subtract 30 seconds from total

## Table 23-3. Off-season Ice Hockey Universal Workout Program

| EXERCISE | PRIMARY MUSCLES DEVELOPED | SPECIFIC SKILLS INVOLVED |
|---|---|---|
| 1. Leg Press* | Buttocks, quadriceps | Skating, checking |
| 2. Leg Extension* | Quadriceps | Skating, checking |
| 3. Leg Curl* | Hamstrings | Skating |
| 4. Bench Press* | Pectorals, deltoids, triceps | Shooting, checking |
| 5. Chin-ups* | Latissimus dorsi, biceps | Shooting, checking |
| 6. Seated Press* | Deltoids, triceps | Shooting |
| 7. Upright Rowing | Deltoids, biceps | Shooting |
| 8. Hyperextension | Lower back | Shooting, skating |
| 9. Triceps Extension | Triceps | Shooting, checking |
| 10. Biceps Curls | Biceps | Checking |
| 11. Wrist Curl* | Forearm flexors | Shooting, gripping stick |
| 12. Reverse Curl | Forearm extensors | Shooting, gripping stick |

*In-season only

- Perform 1 set of 8 to 12 reps of each exercise
- Take no more than 60 seconds to perform each set
- Rest no more than 30 seconds between each set
- To determine *total workout time:* multiply # of workouts by 1½ minutes, then subtract 30 seconds from total

## Table 23-4. Conditioning exercises for ice hockey.

- Use a weight of 10-25 for exercises (1-4)
- Perform all exercises for a minimum of 60 seconds each.
- Gradually increase either the amount of weight used or the length of the exercise bout.

1. "BACKLIFT"
Broadstance, with body bent forward and a slight bending of the knees. The weight lies across the back of the neck, supported by both hands. Stretch briskly and return.

2. "LIFT FROM A LOW POSITION"
Broadstance. Hold the weight with both hands. Swing the weight down backward between the legs at the same time bend the knees slightly. Briskly stretch up (all the way up on your toes) at the same time swing the weight forward and up.

3. "SWING AND BEND WITH THE SACK"
Stand with your legs nearly together. Hold the weight in one hand. Swing the weight back and forth with a bending of the knees. Shift the weight over into the other hand every time that the arm is forward.

4. "EXPLODE"
Stand with the legs a good foot apart, the toes pointing straight forward. The weight lies on the ground close to the legs. Reach down in a relaxed fashion, grip the weight, and "explode" with a strong stretching out and a high lift. Notice: The knees are supposed to be thrust forward at the same time as you reach downward. Concentrate on every single lift.

5. Using a "low duck walk" position with hands and arms on the back, move the body forward while leaning slightly forward with the upper body. To achieve maximum benefit from this exercise, the skater should start a pushing motion early each time he changes the body weight from foot to foot. This exercise is best performed on a slight uphill grade (15°-25°).

# CHAPTER 24
## Judo

Most Judoka recognize five elements as the basic foundations of Judo: knowledge of the sport, speed, timing, balance, and coordination. Each of these components are singularly important and collectively indispensible to Dr. Kano's axiom of maximum efficiency.

In the Dojo, the workouts are generally very similar throughout the country. A workout typically includes: the salutations; calisthenics, warm-up and limbering exercises; Randori; Kata; and Uchikomi. One of the primary considerations of Dr. Kano's original objectives—development of the body—has been virtually ignored in the general Judo practice session. While Judo workouts are, for the most part, very demanding, they do not, however, in themselves, develop the level of fitness required for top flight Judo. The athlete participating in judo must engage in a properly planned conditioning program on a regular basis. The need for additional training can easily be seen in judo matches where after 3 or 4 minutes of the contest both judo players are apparently so fatigued that they appear to be just waltzing around the mat. Such waltzing is the result of both athletes being so exhausted that they can't do anything else! Having attempted their best techniques and having failed, these athletes are simply too tired to continue top flight judo. They have gone from the offensive to a completely defensive posture in an attempt to keep from being thrown to the mat. This lack of fitness ponders Dr. Kano's enlightened analysis that "the ultimate objective of judo is the perfection of one's self by systematic training of the **mind** and **body** through exercise so that each work **in harmony with the other!**"

Successful judo requires a high level of muscular fitness, stamina (cardiovascular fitness), and flexibility. The development of these fitness components should be undertaken on a **year-around** basis. A regular program of weight training (Tables 24-2, 24-3) is the best method for improving muscular fitness. Interval training, in conjunction with a long-slow-distance jogging regimen, is one of the most effective means of developing stamina for judo. Flexibility should also be systematically developed (refer to Chapter 13 of this text).

*The editor is grateful to Roger Capan for his assistance in writing this chapter.

# Judo

## Table 24-1. Judo overview

| BASIC SKILLS | MUSCLES INVOLVED |
|---|---|
| 1. Methods of holding | Flexor pollicis longus, palmaris longus |
| 2. Methods of unbalancing | Flexor digitorum profundus |
| 3. Hand throws | Biceps femoris, rectus abdominus |
| 4. Hip throws | Quadriceps femoris, scalenus |
| 5. Leg throws | Gastroenemus, hamstrings |
| 6. Back and side throws | Deltoids |
| 7. Grappling techniques | Pectoralis |
| 8. Strangling holds | Latissimus dorsi, biceps, deltoids |
| 9. Arm lock techniques | Biceps, triceps, trapezius |

PROBLEM AREAS: After injury failure to recondition properly.

Ankles
Fingers
Neck
Weak shoulders
Wrists
Arms (about the elbow)

*Dislocations and separation of upper extremities
A) Shoulders
B) Elbow
(Could be lessened by stronger torso; arms, shoulders, etc.)

AREAS TO EMPHASIZE:

- Grip strength
- Shoulder strength
- Back strength
- Neck Strength　　　Upper torso of most judoists are weak.
- Stomach muscles
- Legs
- Stamina
- Muscular fatigue
- Emphasize flexibility and joint stability exercises in order to reduce the possibility of injuries

## Table 24-2. Off-season Judo Nautilus Workout Program

| EXERCISE (in order) | PRIMARY MUSCLES DEVELOPED | SPECIFIC SKILLS INVOLVED |
|---|---|---|
| 1. Leg Extension* | Quadriceps | Leg throws & hip throws |
| 2. Leg Press* | Buttocks, major muscles of the legs | Leg throws & hip throws |
| 3. Hip and Back | Buttocks, lower back | Leg throws & Hip throws |
| 4. Leg Curl* | Hamstrings | Leg throws |
| 5. Double Shoulder | Deltoids | Grappling techniques & unbalancing |
| 6. Seated Press | Deltoids, triceps | Grappling techniques & unbalancing |
| 7. Shrugs | Trapezius | Kuzushi — lifting unbalancing |
| 8. Pullover* | Latissimus dorsi | Hip throws, strangling holds unbalancing |
| 9. Chins* | Lats, biceps | Hip throws, strangle holds unbalancing |
| 10. Dips* | Pectorals, deltoids, triceps | Hand throws |
| 11. Biceps Curls | Biceps | Kuzushi — unbalancing (pulling) |
| 12. Wrist Curls | Forearm flexors | Hand throws, Kumikata |
| 13. 4-Way Neck | Neck muscles | Grapping techniques |

*In-season only
- Perform 1 set of 8 to 12 reps of each exercise
- Take no more than 60 seconds to perform each set
- Rest no more than 30 seconds between each set
- To determine **total workout time:** multiply # of workouts by 1½ minutes, then subtract 30 seconds from total.

## Table 24-3. Off-season Judo Universal Workout Program

| EXERCISE (in order) | PRIMARY MUSCLES DEVELOPED | SPECIFIC SKILLS INVOLVED |
|---|---|---|
| 1. Leg Press* | Buttocks, major muscles of the legs | Leg throws & hip throws |
| 2. Leg Extension* | Quadriceps | Leg throws & hip throws |
| 3. Leg Curl* | Hamstrings | Leg throws |
| 4. Bench Press* | Pectorals, deltoids, triceps | Grappling techniques |
| 5. Chinups* | Lats, biceps | Hip throws, strangling holds — unbalancing, Kumikata |
| 6. Seated Press | Deltoids, triceps | Grappling techniques |
| 7. Lat Pulldown | Lats, biceps | Hand throws, Kumikata |
| 8. Hyperextension | Lower back | Hip throws & leg throws |
| 9. Dips* | Pectorals, deltoids, triceps | Hand throws |
| 10. Biceps Curls | Biceps | Kuzushi — unbalancing (pulling) |
| 11. Wrist Curls | Forearm flexors | Hand throws, Kumikata |
| 12. Neck Exercises | Neck muscles | Grappling techniques |

*In-season only
- Perform 1 set of 8 to 12 reps of each exercise
- Take no more than 60 seconds to perform each set
- Rest no more than 30 seconds between each set
- To determine **total workout time:** multiply # of workouts by 1½ minutes, then subtract 30 seconds from total.

# CHAPTER 25
## Lacrosse

Proficiency in the sport of lacrosse requires a high level of **total** fitness and a mastery of a wide variety of skills. Skill improvement is best achieved through a combination of competent coaching and dedicated practice. Fitness is most effectively developed by adherence to the principles and techniques articulated in Chapter 1-13.

Lacrosse requires that the athlete possess stamina, muscular fitness, flexibility and an extensive array of motor abilities. Adequate stamina enables the individual to meet the cardiovascular demands imposed by this fast-moving sport. Muscular fitness has an effect on almost every aspect of lacrosse—shooting, stick control, body checking, running, and (perhaps most importantly) preventing muscular fatigue. Since flexibility and joint stability play an important role in the success of a lacrosse player, improvement in these factors should be given adequate attention in every lacrosseman's conditioning program. Such attention, not only will affect the lacrosseman's performance on the field, but will also decrease his possibility of incurring an injury.

*The editor is grateful to Major Al Girardi for his assistance in writing this chapter.

Table 25-1. Lacrosse overview

| BASIC SKILLS | MUSCLES INVOLVED |
|---|---|
| 1. Body checking | Buttocks, lower back, quadriceps, hamstrings |
| 2. Stick checking | Pectorals, deltoids, triceps, biceps, latissimus dorsi |
| 3. Shooting | Latissimus dorsi, deltoids, triceps, biceps, pectorals |
| 4. Cradling | Forearm flexors, latissimus dorsi, deltoids, triceps, biceps, pectorals |

PROBLEM AREAS:

Stamina
Muscular fatigue
Grip strength
Knee and shoulder injuries

AREAS TO EMPHASIZE:

- Develop the musculature used in lacrosse to prevent muscular fatigue
- Develop the hand and forearm flexors to ensure adequate grip strength
- Emphasize exercises for joint stability and flexibility in order to reduce the possibility of injuries
- Develop stamina by extensive work using a combination interval training, circuit training, and/or prolonged jogging
- Warm-up properly

## Table 25-2 Off-season Lacrosse Nautilus Workout Program

| EXERCISE (in order) | PRIMARY MUSCLES DEVELOPED | SPECIFIC SKILLS INVOLVED |
|---|---|---|
| 1. Hip and Back* | Buttocks, Lower back* | Body and stick checking |
| 2. Leg Extension* | Quadriceps | Running, cutting |
| 3. Leg Press | Buttocks, quadriceps | Running, cutting |
| 4. Leg Curl* | Hamstrings | Running, cutting |
| 5. Double Chest (fly movement) | Pectorals | Cradling, shooting |
| 6. Double Chest (decline press) | Pectorals, deltoids, triceps | Checking, shooting cradling |
| 7. Pullover* | Latissimus dorsi | Checking, shooting, cradling |
| 8. Torso Arm* | Latissimus dorsi, biceps | Shooting, cradling |
| 9. Dips* | Pectorals, deltoids, triceps | Face-offs, cradling, shooting |
| 10. Biceps Curls* | Biceps | Face-offs, cradling, shooting |
| 11. Triceps Extension* | Triceps | Face-offs, cradling, shooting |
| 12. Wrist Curls* | Forearm Flexors | Face-offs, cradling, shooting |

- Perform 1 set of 8 to 12 reps of each exercise
- Take no more than 60 seconds to perform each set
- Rest no more than 30 seconds between each set
- To determine **total workout time:** multiply # of workouts by 1½ minutes, then subtract 30 seconds from total

*In-season only

## Table 25-3. Off-season Lacrosse Universal Workout Program

| EXERCISE (in order) | PRIMARY MUSCLES DEVELOPED | SPECIFIC SKILLS INVOLVED |
|---|---|---|
| 1. Leg Press* | Buttocks, quadriceps | Running, checking, cutting |
| 2. Leg Extension | Quadriceps | Running, checking, cutting |
| 3. Leg Curl* | Hamstrings | Running, checking, cutting |
| 4. Bench Press* | Pectorals, deltoids, triceps | Face-offs, shooting, cradling |
| 5. Lat. Pulldown | Latissimus dorsi, biceps | Shooting, cradling, checking |
| 6. Seated Press* | Deltoids, triceps | Shooting, cradling, checking |
| 7. Upright Rowing | Deltoids, biceps | Shooting, cradling, checking |
| 8. Hyperextension* | Lower back | Checking, running, cutting |
| 9. Shrug* | Trapezius | Checking, cradling |
| 10. Tricep Extension* | Triceps | Shooting, cradling, face-offs |
| 11. Biceps Curls* | Biceps | Shooting, cradling, face-offs |
| 12. Wrist Curls* | Forearm Flexors | Shooting, cradling, face-offs |

- Perform 1 set of 8 to 12 reps of each exercise
- Take no more than 60 seconds to perform each set
- Rest no more than 30 seconds between each set
- To determine **total workout time:** multiply # of workouts by 1½ minutes, then subtract 30 seconds from total

*In-season only

# CHAPTER 26
## Racquetball

Racquetball is a fast moving, high intensity, physically demanding activity. Speed of movement, explosive power, hand-eye coordination and the ability to maintain these attributes at a high level during the course of a match are essential skills of the successful racquetballer. Conditioning for racquetball, therefore, encompasses sharpening (improving) the following factors: endurance, strength, speed and agility, flexibility, and coordination. While playing the game itself is probably the best "overall" conditioner for the racquetballer, a properly planned conditioning program should augment the time spent in the court playing.

Running should be included in any conditioning program for racquetball. Depending on the athlete's devotion to the game, the conditioning regimen will vary from a few long distance runs of 2-3 miles to a demanding program combining distance runs, interval work and sprint workouts. The long runs are included to develop the aerobic capacity required to play those extended 3-game matches, while the sprint training helps develop the quickness needed for explosive movements about the court. The interval work benefits both speed and endurance. Skipping rope and Stauffer's Star Drill should also be included in the running program in order to improve quickness and agility.

All conditioning routines should include some form of stretching or flexibility exercises. Racquetball is **no** exception. Increased flexibility will not only improve the athlete's on-the-court performance, but will also improve his chances of avoiding injuries. Before and after both workouts and games are the best times to stretch or loosen up. Of particular concern to the racquetballer are the muscles of the legs, lower back, and racquet arm. Flexibility exercises need by no more elaborate than toe or straddle stretches and leg pullovers from the supine position, but they should be of the static stretch variety in which the muscles and joints are loosened by the individual's body weight, not by bouncing movements.

Muscular development is essential both to a racquetballer's overall performance in a court and to help prevent injuries. The player deficient in muscular fitness will normally observe a gradual reduction in his performance level during the course of a prolonged match or tournament. Development of strength in the muscles used to run and to hit the ball helps to prevent or minimize injury to such areas as the knees,

*The editor is grateful to Captain Jed Cantlay for his assistance in writing this chapter.

shoulders, and the elbow of the dominant arm. In addition, greater strength increases the athlete's ability to move quickly and to hit with power.

No two racquetball players are alike. A conditioning program that aids one individual may not necessarily affect another athlete as much. In order to "personalize" his conditioning program, the individual player should use the program planning principles articulated in Chapter 13. Such a program will enable the athlete to achieve a level of fitness which will permit the best possible level of performance.

Table 26-1. Racquetball overview

| BASIC SKILLS | MUSCLES INVOLVED |
|---|---|
| 1. Running, cutting movements | Buttocks, lower back, quadriceps, hamstrings |
| 2. Hitting the ball | Pectorals, triceps, biceps, latissimus dorsi |
| 3. Wrist control | Hand and forearm flexors |

PROBLEM AREAS:

Stamina
Muscular fatigue
Grip strength
Elbow and shoulder injuries

AREAS TO EMPHASIZE:

- Implement an aerobic program for stamina

- Develop the musculature involved in racquetball to prevent muscular fatigue

- Emphasize joint stability and flexibility exercises in order to reduce the possibility of injuries

- Develop grip strength to improve racquet control

- Warm-up properly

## Table 26-2. Racquetball Nautilus Workout Program*

| EXERCISE (in order) | PRIMARY MUSCLES DEVELOPED | SPECIFIC SKILLS INVOLVED |
|---|---|---|
| 1. Leg Extension | Quadriceps | Running |
| 2. Leg Press | Buttocks, quadriceps | Running |
| 3. Hip and Back | Buttocks | Running, hitting the ball |
| 4. Leg Curl | Hamstring | Running |
| 5. Double Shoulder (lateral raise) | Deltoids | Hitting the ball, prevent shoulder injuries |
| 6. Double Shoulder (seated press) | Deltoids, triceps | Hitting the ball, prevent shoulder injuries |
| 7. Pullover | Latissimus dorsi | Hitting the ball |
| 8. Biceps Curls | Biceps | Pronating the forearm when hitting the ball, prevent hyperextension of the elbow |
| 9. Triceps Extension | Triceps | Hitting the ball, follow thru, prevent elbow injuries |
| 10. Wrist Curl | Forearm Flexors | Gripping the racquet, wrist control |
| 11. Squeeze a Rubber Ball | Hand flexors | Gripping the racquet, wrist control |

- Perform 1 set of 8 to 12 reps of each exercise
- Take no more than 60 seconds to perform each set
- Rest no more than 30 seconds between each set
- To determine **total workout time:** multiply # of workouts by 1½ minutes, then subtract 30 seconds from total

*Since for most individuals racquetball is a year-around activity, the frequency of this program should be adjusted to meet the individual situation.

## Table 26-3. Racquetball Universal Workout Program*

| EXERCISE (in order) | PRIMARY MUSCLES DEVELOPED | SPECIFIC SKILLS INVOLVED |
|---|---|---|
| 1. Leg Press | Buttocks, quadriceps | Running |
| 2. Leg Extension | Quadriceps | Running |
| 3. Leg Curl | Hamstrings | Running |
| 4. Bench Press | Pectorals, deltoids, triceps | Hitting the ball, prevent shoulder and elbow injuries |
| 5. Lat Pulldown | Latissimus dorsi, biceps | Hitting the ball |
| 6. Seated Press | Deltoids, triceps | Hitting the ball, minimize shoulder and elbow injuries |
| 7. Upright Rowing | Deltoids, biceps | Hitting the ball |
| 8. Triceps Extension | Triceps | Hitting the ball and follow thru, prevent elbow injuries |
| 9. Biceps Curls | Biceps | Hitting the ball |
| 10. Wrist Curls | Forearm flexors | Wrist control, gripping the racquet |
| 11. Squeeze a Rubber Ball | Hand flexors | Wrist control, gripping the racquet |

- Perform 1 set of 8 to 12 reps of each exercise ·
- Take no more than 60 seconds to perform each set
- Rest no more than 30 seconds between each set
- To determine **total workout time:** multiply # of workouts by 1½ minutes, then subtract 30 seconds from total

*Since for most individuals, racquetball is a year-around activity, the frequency of this program should be adjusted to meet the individual situation.

# Racquetball

## Table 26-4. A sample conditioning schedule for racquetball*

A. Off-Season

| M, W, F | T, Th, S | S |
|---|---|---|
| Stretch | Strength Dev. | Rest |

Run 2-6 miles
depending on individual)

Play racquetball whenever desired. Building the conditioning base is most important during this phase. When playing, work on new shots and have fun in the court—do not get "stale" or bored with the game.

B. Pre-Season (6 weeks before tournament play)

| M, F | T, Th | W, S | Sun |
|---|---|---|---|
| Stretch/Warm-up | Same as M, F | Stretch | Rest |
| *Drills in court | except substitute | Games (60 min.) | |
| Games (30-60 min) | Str Dev for Run | Jog 1 mile, | |
| Run-jog ¼ mile | Skip rope 5 min | 2-3 on Sat | |
| run 10/50 yd | | | |
| sprints | | | |
| 15-30 sec | | | |
| between | | | |
| sprints | | | |
| jog ¼ mile | | | |

*including 2 Star Drills

C. In-Season (Tournaments, usually on the weekends)

| M, W | T | Th |
|---|---|---|
| Stretch/Warm-up | Stretch, Warm-up | Rest |
| Drills (60 min) | Easy games (30-60 min) | |
| Run-jog ¼ mile | Easy 2 mile jog | |
| 10/50 yd sprints | Strength Workout | |
| (5 on Wed) | | |
| jog ¼ mile | | |
| Skip rope 5 min | | |

*These workouts may be too ambitious for the player whose time is limited. On the other hand, a serious devotee of the game may spend more time and effort in conditioning.

# CHAPTER 27
## Rugby

Modern rugby is a mixture of both complex and specialized skills, placing great physical demands on the body. As one of the world's most rigorous and fast moving activities, rugby has enjoyed a rapid increase in the number of both participants and spectators.

Considerable differences exist in the United States as to the game's approach. Geography (climate), number of competitive seasons played by a team during the year, and the number of training sessions per week (team or individual) are a few of the pertinent variables which must be considered when formulating a fitness program for rugby. This chapter is organized to provide guidelines for the development of conditioning programs for rugby which are applicable to any situation.

### PHYSICAL COMPONENTS OF THE RUGBY PLAYER

The following fitness-related components are essential to successful rugby: endurance, strength (to include explosive power and speed), agility, flexibility, and cardiovascular fitness. The necessity for a high level of muscular fitness is vital if for no other reason than injury prevention. Numerous late season injuries could undoubtedly be avoided by a properly planned off season muscular development program.

Because rugby involves continuous slow-fast running by the ruggers almost the entire length of a match (particularly by the forward), rugby players must possess a high level of cardiovascular fitness. A more efficient heart and lungs will enable the athlete to recover more quickly from demands imposed by the numerous short, maximal bouts of work which occur during a match.

### PHASE ONE: OFF-SEASON TRAINING

This phase extends from the end of the competitive season until roughly eight weeks prior to the next season. In concept, conditioning and training should be relatively less vigorous than the physical demands of match competition. The main emphasis should be on building a substantial base of muscular and cardiovascular fitness. Such a base must be developed **prior** to the 6-8 weeks before the season begins so that the athlete can concentrate on sharpening his skills and level of fitness immediately before the start of the season.

Flexibility exercises should also be an integral part of the off-season conditioning program for rugby. The pressure that is exerted on the shoulder joints of the props and hookers when a scrum collapses is one

*The editor is grateful to Captain Robert Hensler for his assistance in writing this chapter.

of the most vivid examples of the need for **flexibility** and **joint stability** for rugby players.

A typical weekly off-season conditioning program for rugby would include the following: strength training on Monday, Wednesday and Friday; aerobic conditioning (e.g. running, handball, racquetball, basketball, etc) on Tuesday, Thursday and Sunday; and relaxation on Sunday. While running is unquestionably the best developer of cardio-vascular fitness, other larger muscle activities should be incorporated into the conditioning program in order to give variety to the training program.

## PHASE TWO: PRE-SEASON TRAINING

Preseason training (the six to eight weeks preceding actual competition) should reflect two main conditioning principles: *specificity and overload*. Specificity for rugby involves training at match or near-match intensity and concentrating on skills (passing, kicking, rucking, etc.) specific to the position played. Overload simply means placing sufficient demands on the body to bring about improved fitness. While all properly planned conditioning involves the overload principle, the greatest degree of overload should occur during preseason training.

Having established an adequate aerobic base in the offseason, the athlete should now attempt to develop anaerobic or match fitness. Rugby, particularly forward play, is a continuous series of short, very exhaustive bouts of work, demanding anaerobic energy (refer to Chapter 2 for a more extension discussion of aerobic vs anaerobic work). The rugger (depending on his position) needs to possess sufficient anaerobic energy capacity to perform multiple sprints with relief coming only as the athlete jogs back into position. The forwards, for example, engage in multiple repetitions of short, very intense bouts of work lasting up to 20 seconds (rucks/mouls) with intermittent periods of jogging between work efforts (corner flogging, following scrums, rucks, etc.).

A sample weekly workout schedule for rugby during the preseason would include the following: strength training on Monday, Wednesday, and Friday; fast interval work (3-4 miles) on Tuesday; acceleration sprints (1.5 miles) on Thursday; fartlek training (3-4 miles) on Saturday, and rest on Sunday. The intensity of the aforementioned workouts can be modified by varying the amount of distance run.

For *optimum development of match fitness* the training time during interval work should be approximately 60 seconds per interval. The length of the interval should vary as the situation dictates. The usual distances employed in interval work are 110's, 220's, 440's *and* half miles.

Whenever feasible, match skills should also be developed during the preseason. Much of the running program should be accompanied by the passing/kicking of a ball. Touch rugby is another excellent method to not only warm-up, but also practice passing techniques.

## PHASE THREE: IN-SEASON TRAINING

All ruggers should be in a high state of physical readiness *before* competition begins. Training at this time should be almost totally *match oriented*. Running of any kind should be accompanied by ball passing, kicking, dribbling, slipping, etc. The major objective of training, should be improvement of individual and team skills, developing tactics and team unity, and maintaining match fitness.

## PRACTICE

Each practice session should be organized as efficiently as possible. The less standing around, talking about "how to", the better results the practice will achieve.

Some individuals argue that physical fitness is the individual's responsibility and that practice time should not be "wasted" on physical training. Such an opinion is totally without merit. Fitness development *can* and *should* be integrated into the practice session. For example, most clubs, particularly at the beginning of their season, spend time on individual and unit skills. The following 7-step practice drill illustrates how *both* fitness and skill may be enhanced by means of basic ball handling drills. For this drill, both backs and forwards can be intermixed since the basic skills should be mastered by both positions.

1. Groups of 3-6 players are placed in grids roughly 15 x 15 meters. The width of the field is not important. Accuracy and quickness of handling are stressed.

2. Players pass the ball to one another going back and forth in the grid as rapidly as possible. Passing should be performed in all directions. Accuracy is stressed initially with the speed of the pass increased as accuracy improves.

3. Dribbling and grub kicking are added along with picking up the loose ball.

4. The individual picking up the ball either executes a quick feed pass or, using the attacking fall, flips the ball up based on knowledge of his teammates' location.

5. "Shadow" mauling and rucking follow with one player used to "resist".

6. Ball stripping with continued mauling/rucking follows. The group

should be evenly divided between attackers and defenders.

7. Form tackling is next introduced with emphasis on creating the maul or ruck with feeding, and skipping leading to continued possession by the attackers.

The aforementioned 7-step drill involves most of the individual skills required of all players. The back, for example, who can not create the ruck when tackled is of marginal value. Performing this drill for 10-15 minutes will overload the cardiovascular system thereby developing player stamina. The concentration required to properly execute this drill, especially as fatigue sets in, should lead to improved player discipline. The major points to stress are: precision of execution; continuous action; and minimum discussion (learn by example).

Probably the best way to end practice is with a brisk game of unopposed rugby. Movement to the ball should be at maximum pace. Wings should create the maul upon receipt of the ball. Coaches should vigorously extol the forwards to push themselves. This technique not only promotes fitness but also is beneficial for developing player discipline under stress.

# Rugby

## Table 27-1. Rugby overview

| BASIC SKILLS | MUSCLES INVOLVED |
|---|---|
| 1. Rucking/scrum | Buttocks, quadriceps, hamstrings, lower back |
| 2. Tackling | Pectorals, deltoids, triceps, biceps, latissimus dorsi, neck flexors and extensors, trapezius |
| 3. Passing the ball | Latissimus dorsi, deltoids, biceps, pectorals |
| 4. Kicking | Buttocks, quadriceps, illiopsoas, lower back |
| 5. Running | Buttocks, quadriceps, hamstrings, lower back |

PROBLEM AREAS:

> Stamina
> Muscular fatigue
> Shoulder injuries
> Neck strength

AREAS TO EMPHASIZE:

- Develop stamina by means of a variety of the aerobic programs described in Chapters 8 and 13.

- Develop the musculature involved in rugby to prevent muscular fatigue.

- Emphasize flexibility and joint stability exercises to minimize the possibility of injuries

- Develop the neck musculature to meet the extensive demands imposed on the neck during the scrum

- Warm-up properly.

## Table 27-2. Off-season Rugby Nautilus Workout Program

| EXERCISE (in order) | PRIMARY MUSCLES DEVELOPED | SPECIFIC SKILLS INVOLVED |
|---|---|---|
| 1. Hip and back* | Buttocks | Scrum, running, jumping, rucking, kicking |
| 2. Leg Extension* | Quadriceps | Scrum, running, jumping, rucking, kicking |
| 3. Leg Press | Buttocks, quadriceps | Scrum, rucking, kicking, running, jumping |
| 4. Leg Curl* | Hamstrings | Running |
| 5. Double Chest* (bent arm fly) | Pectorals | Scrum, hitting, tackling, rucking |
| 6. Double Chest (decline press) | Pectorals, deltoids, triceps | Scrum, rucking, hitting, tackling, throwing |
| 7. Pullover* | Latissimus dorsi, biceps | Catching ball and pulling to the chest, throwing |
| 8. Chin-ups | Latissimus dorsi, biceps | Catching ball and pulling to the chest, throwing |
| 9. Dips* | Pectorals, deltoids, triceps | Scrum, rucking, hitting, tackling |
| 10. Biceps Curls | Biceps | Hold ball while running, tackling |
| 11. 4-way Neck* | Neck flexors and extensors | Scrum, rucking, tackling |
| 12. Shrug | Trapezius | Scrum, rucking, tackling |

- Perform 1 set of 8 to 12 reps of each exercise
- Take no more than 60 seconds to perform each set
- Rest no more than 30 seconds between each set
- To determine **total workout time:** multiply # of workouts by 1½ minutes, then subtract 30 seconds from total

*In-season only

## Table 27-3. Off-season Rugby Universal Workout Program

| EXERCISE<br>(in order) | PRIMARY MUSCLES<br>DEVELOPED | SPECIFIC SKILLS<br>INVOLVED |
|---|---|---|
| 1. Leg Press* | Buttocks, quadriceps | Scrum, rucking, kicking, running, jumping, tackling |
| 2. Leg Extension | Quadriceps | Scrum, rucking, running, kicking, jumping, tackling |
| 3. Leg Curl* | Hamstrings | Running |
| 4. Bench Press* | Pectorals, deltoids, triceps | Scrum, rucking, tacling, throwing |
| 5. Lat Pulldown* | Latissimus dorsi, biceps | Throwing |
| 6. Seated Press | Deltoids, triceps | Scrum, rucking, tackling, throwing |
| 7. Upright Row | Deltoids, biceps | Scrum, rucking, tackling |
| 8. Hyperextension* | Lower back | Set scrums, loose play |
| 9. Shrug | Trapezius | Scrum, tackling, hitting, supporting neck |
| 10. Dips* | Pectorals, deltoids, triceps | Tackling, hitting, throwing |
| 11. Biceps Curls | Biceps | Tackling, hitting, hold ball while running |
| 12. Neck Station* | Neck flexors, extensors | Support neck, tackling, scrums |

- Perform 1 set of 8 to 12 reps of each exercise
- Take no more than 60 seconds to perform each set
- Rest no more than 30 seconds between each set
- To determine **total workout time:** multiply # of workouts by 1½ minutes, then subtract 30 seconds from total

*In-season only

## Table 27-4. Year-around conditioning schedule for rugby.

**END OF SEASON**
(BEGINNING OF OFF
SEASON TRAINING)

**PRESEASON** (6-8 WEEKS
PRIOR TO COMPETITION)

**INSEASON**
LENGTH VARIES IN
DIFFERENT LOCATIONS

### OFFSEASON

General body conditioning (remaining
physically active)

**Strength Trng** — 3 times/wk — all major
muscle groups

***Endurance Trng** — Aerobic

long duration
submaximal intensity
long slow distance running
slow interval
continuous fast running
interval sprints
indoor/outdoor court games
swimming
cycling

**Flexibility trng.**
slow deliberate/static stretching before
and after training

**Match skills**
Individual skills

**Self testing**

**Intensity** — generally lower than
competition

*See Chapter 2 for explanation of terms.
These are a few of the items that may be
incorporated into a program.

### PRESEASON

Keys are **specificity** and **overload** —
training intensity, work intervals should be
as close as possible to match pace

**Strength training** — 3 times/wk all major
muscle groups

**Endurance training** — Anaerobic
*(match intensity)
jog-sprints
acceleration sprints
fast interval
Fartlek
Repetition running

**Flexibility** same as preseason

**Match skills** — last 3-4 wks
concentrate on doing all training with a
ball and other players. Work on individual
and unit skills

### INSEASON

All training is done to improve directly
skills involved in playing rugby.
i.e., intensity and duration are identical to
match situations. Fitness training should,
for best results, be done with a ball
approximating competition.

Unopposed rugby — excellent method of
combining skills and fitness training.

**Strength training** — 2 times/wk

**Endurance** — Anaerobic

**Flexibility** — same as off- and pre-season.

# CHAPTER 28
## Skiing

Skiing is undoubtedly one of the most demanding sports, mentally and physically, that the average individual ever takes up. Certainly athletes can decide on the effort they expend towards skiing. They can miss a good ski run or go slower down the slope or sit in the sun all afternoon discussing turns at the ski lodge. By the same token individuals will increase their enjoyment of even a modest ski holiday if they engage in a properly planned program of conditioning prior to taking to the slopes. Although some skiers may feel that such an expenditure of effort is wasteful, the benefits of improved fitness far outweigh the energy cost of achieving such improvement.

While individuals can still enjoy skiing without any major program of pre-season conditioning, skiers need not have the irritating aches and pains which frequently result from a day on the ski slope; individuals need not endanger themselves by skiing closer to their physical limits than is safe; and skiees probably would be more proficient at the end of their initial ski outings if they had prepared for them. Think of it this way: a get-fit pre-season program takes half-hours at home but adds hours of skiing to the normal skiing holiday. An individual may tell himself that he is already adequately fit. Self-deception! Skiing will detect and work muscles that the average individual did not know were there. Conditioning for skiing should emphasize the development of two components of fitness: flexibility and muscular fitness.

The pre-season conditioning program for skiing should be started 5-6 weeks before the ski season begins. The individual who starts pre-season conditioning the week before the season merely arrives at the ski slope with muscle aches already in hand.

The pre-season program should not concentrate only on muscular development. Flexibility exercises are required as well as exercises for strength and endurance. An athlete who ignores the development of an adequate level of flexibility will not be prepared for the numerous twists and turns involved in skiing.

The muscles that are most important to skiing are those of the legs that produce the side-to-side and rotating movements required to initiate turns. When these muscles do not have an adequate level of development (particularly at the beginning of the season), the skier is frequently forced to utilize a pivitol movement of the hips or the upper-body to start his skis turning. This adjustment not only makes for a

*The editor is grateful to Major Robert Frank for his assistance in writing this chapter.

delayed turn, it also keeps the individual's skiing pleasure to a minimum because he does not have total, confident control of his skis. Consequently, it is obvious that the time spent in the exercise room will reward the skier many times over by allowing the individual to start his ski season prepared for challenges of the slope.

---

Table 28-1. Skiing overview

| BASIC SKILLS | MUSCLES INVOLVED |
|---|---|
| 1. Maintain weight over skis | Quadriceps, hamstrings, buttocks |
| 2. Absorb shock of landings | Quadriceps, hamstrings, buttocks |
| 3. Driving off poles | Deltoids, triceps, latissimus dorsi |
| 4. Maintain balance | Quadriceps, hamstrings, lower back |

PROBLEM AREAS:

Muscular endurance
Stamina
Knee injuries
Ankle injuries

AREAS TO EMPHASIZE:

- Develop musculature involved in the basis skills of skiing

- Develop stamina using a comprehensive running/interval training

- Develop joint stability through strength conditioning of muscles surrounding susceptible joints

- Emphasis extensive flexibility conditioning

## Table 28-2. Pre-season Skiing Nautilus Workout Program

| EXERCISE (in order) | PRIMARY MUSCLES DEVELOPED | SPECIFIC SKILLS INVOLVED |
|---|---|---|
| 1. Hip and Back* | Buttocks, lower back | Maintain weight over skis, maintain balance, absorb shock on landings |
| 2. Leg Extension* | Quadriceps | Absorbing shock on landing, maintain weight over skis |
| 3. Leg Press* | Buttocks, quadriceps | Maintain balance, absorb shock on landings, maintain weight over skis |
| 4. Leg Curl* | Hamstrings | Stabilizes legs and knee joint, maintain balance |
| 5. Double Shoulder (lateral raise) | Deltoids | Extending arms, driving off poles, forward arm swing |
| 6. Double Shoulder* (seated press) | Deltoids, triceps | Driving off poles, arm extension |
| 7. Pullover* | Latissimus dorsi | Driving off poles, maneuvering into position |
| 8. Torso-arm | Latissimus dorsi, biceps | Stabilize elbow joint |
| 9. Triceps extension | Triceps | Extending arms |
| 10. Wrist Curls* | Forearm flexors | Grip strength for holding poles |

- Perform 1 set of 8 to 12 reps of each exercise during off-season
- Take no more than 60 seconds to perform each set
- Rest no more than 30 seconds between each set
- To determine **total workout time:** multiply # of workouts by 1½ minutes, then subtract 30 seconds from total

*In-season only

## Table 28-3. Pre-season Skiing Universal Workout Program

| EXERCISE (in order) | PRIMARY MUSCLES DEVELOPED | SPECIFIC SKILLS INVOLVED |
|---|---|---|
| 1. Leg Press* | Buttocks, quadriceps | Maintain weight over skis, maintain balance, absorb shock on landings |
| 2. Leg extension* | Quadriceps | Absorb shock on landings, maintain balance |
| 3. Leg Curl* | Hamstrings | Stabilize legs and knee joint |
| 4. Seated Press* | Deltoids, triceps | Arm extension, driving off plates |
| 5. Upright Rowing | Deltoids, biceps | Driving off poles, stabilize elbow joint |
| 6. Hyperextension | Lower back | Maintaining balance, maintain weight over skis |
| 7. Dips* | Pectorals, deltoids, triceps | Driving off poles, extending the arms |
| 8. Lat Pulldown* | Latissimus dorsi, biceps | Driving off poles |
| 9. Triceps extension* | Triceps | Arm extension |
| 10. Wrist Curl* | Forearm flexors | Grip strength for holding poles |

- Perform 1 set of 8 to 12 reps of each exercise during the season
- Take no more than 60 seconds to perform each set
- Rest no more than 30 seconds between each set
- To determine **total workout time:** multiply # of workouts by 1½ minutes, then subtract 30 seconds from total
- *In-season only

# CHAPTER 29
## Soccer

Soccer is a sport which requires "total fitness" of its participants. Played by both *men* and *women* the world over, soccer is a fast moving game involving stamina, muscular fitness, flexibility, motor skills, and the ability to make instantaneous, accurate decisions. Depending on the position of the player, the game involves almost continuous movement. As a result, an adequate level of cardiovascular fitness is an absolute necessity. Such stamina can best be developed by means of one of the numerous programs for aerobic conditioning discussed in Chapters 8 and 13.

Muscular fitness is important to the soccer player for a number of reasons. For example, a high level of leg strength is an essential component of "kicking power"—a vital skill in soccer. Well-developed neck musculature is required for "heading" the ball. In addition, highly proficient soccer players usually possess well-developed abdomen and trunk muscles.

Other fitness-related factors also play an important role in "successful soccer." Flexibility and joint stability, for example, contribute both to performance improvement and to a general reduction in the possibility of incurring injuries. A higher level of fitness also has a positive influence in selected motor abilities.

*The editor is grateful to Captain Mike Spinello for his assistance in writing this chapter.

## Table 29-1. Soccer overview

| BASIC SKILLS | MUSCLES INVOLVED |
|---|---|
| 1. Kicking | Buttocks, quadriceps, lower back, gastroenemius |
| 2. Heading the ball | Trapezius, neck extensors and flexors |
| 3. Running | Buttocks, hamstrings, quadriceps, lower back |

PROBLEM AREAS:
Stamina
Muscular fatigue
Lower leg injuries
Neck injuries

AREAS TO EMPHASIZE:
- Develop stamina (wind) by engaging in an extensive aerobic conditioning program
- Develop the musculature involved in soccer by an overall muscle fitness program in order to prevent muscular fatigue
- Emphasize the neck and lower legs in the muscle development program in order to minimize the possibility of injuries
- Emphasize flexibility and joint stability exercises
- Warm-up properly

## Table 29-2. Sample circuit training programs for soccer.

| I.  BASIC CIRCUIT FOR SOCCER SKILLS | II.  BASIC CIRCUIT FOR STAMINA |
|---|---|
| a. Sprint 20 yards and then jump to head a soccer ball suspended in the air. | a. 100 yard of fartlek training (sprint, jog, sprint, jog, etc.) |
| b. Dribble a ball around a course delineated by pylons. | b. Run and cut through a pre-marked course. |
| c. Perform throw-ins by use of a heavy ball (e.g. medicine ball), aim at a target above the ground. | c. 25 yards of sprinting backwards. |
| d. Dribble 20 yards, push pass the against an obstacle, collect the rebound, return by dribbling the ball to the starting line. | d. Sprint 10 yards forward, then 10 yards laterally; repeat 5 times. |
| e. "Chip" pass the ball over an obstacle to a partner who controls the ball and repeats. | e. Sprint 100 yards at 3/4 pace, kicking a ball placed every 10 yards to predetermined varying directions. |

## Table 29-3. Off-season Soccer Nautilus Workout Program

| EXERCISE (in order) | PRIMARY MUSCLES DEVELOPED | SPECIFIC SKILLS INVOLVED |
| --- | --- | --- |
| 1. Leg Extension* | Quadriceps | Running, jumping, kicking |
| 2. Leg Press | Buttocks, quadriceps | Running, jumping, kicking |
| 3. Hip and Back* | Buttocks, lower back | Running, jumping, kicking |
| 4. Leg Curl* | Hamstrings | Running |
| 5. Heel Raises* | Calves | Running, kicking, stabilize ankle |
| 6. Double Shoulder* (lateral raise) | Deltoids | Hitting, prevent injury |
| 7. Double Shoulder (seated press) | Deltoids, triceps | Hitting, prevent injury |
| 8. Shrug* | Trapezius | Head the ball |
| 9. Pullover* | Latissimus dorsi | Strengthen back, increase shoulder, flexibility, prevent injury |
| 10. 4-Way Neck* | Neck flexors, extensors | Head the ball |
| 11. Wrist Curl | Forearm flexors | Grip strength (for goalie only) |

- Perform 1 set of 8 to 12 reps of each exercise
- Take no more than 60 seconds to perform each set
- Rest no more than 30 seconds between each set
- To determine **total workout time:** multiply # of workouts by 1½ minutes, then subtract 30 seconds from total

*In-season only

## Table 29-4. Off-season Soccer Universal Workout Program

| EXERCISE (in order) | PRIMARY MUSCLES DEVELOPED | SPECIFIC SKILLS INVOLVED |
|---|---|---|
| 1. Leg Press | Buttocks, quadriceps | Jumping, running, kicking |
| 2. Leg Extension* | Quadriceps | Jumping, running, kicking |
| 3. Leg Curl* | Hamstrings | Running |
| 4. Heel Raises* | Calves | Jumping, running, kicking |
| 5. Seated Press* | Deltoids, triceps | Hitting, prevent injuries |
| 6. Upright Rowing* | Deltoids, biceps | Hitting, prevent injuries |
| 8. Neck Station* | Neck flexors, extensors | |
| 7. Shrug* | Trapezius | Head the ball |
| 8. Neck Station* | Neck flexors, extensors | Head the ball |
| 9. Wrist Curl | Forearm flexors | Grip strength (for goalie only) |

*In-season only
- Perform 1 set of 8 to 12 reps of each exercise
- Take no more than 60 seconds to perform each set
- Rest no more than 30 seconds between each set
- To determine **total workout time:** multiply # of workouts by 1½ minutes, then subtract 30 seconds from total.

# CHAPTER 30
## Swimming

The swimmer should be concerned with all of the basic components of physical fitness: muscular fitness, cardiovascular fitness, flexibility and body composition. Strength and flexibility are most efficiently improved by means of conditioning exercises "out-of-the-water" while cardiovascular fitness and muscular endurance for swimming are most easily achieved through "in-the-water-work."

Although the swimmer utilizes a wider variety of muscle groups than do many athletes, a conditioning program for swimming should concentrate on those muscles which are the "prime movers" in the water. Swimmers are propelled through the water by two major methods: leg action and arm pull. A swimmer can produce his greatest forward thrust when leaving the starting block and when pushing off from a turn. As a result, a muscular development program for swimming should include exercises for the leg extensors—the quadriceps, the gastroenemius, and the gluteal muscles.

In all of the four major competitive strokes the arm pull is the primary source of propulsion through the water. Consequently, the swimmer's weight training program should include exercises for the development of the triceps, the latissimus dorsi, the pectorals, and the teres major. In addition, the inward rotations of the arm, the wrist flexors, and the elbow extensors should be properly developed. In many instances, these latter muscle groups are frequently ignored in the swimmer's training regimen.

Muscular endurance should be developed through long hours of water work. Such effort will also contribute somewhat to the athlete's attempts to control his level of body fat. Interval training and circuit training are two of the best programs for cardiovascular fitness improvement.

Flexibility is also important—particularly of the shoulder and ankle joints. Forced stretching, by means of working in pairs on the pool deck, is one of the most effective techniques for developing flexibility. Several "paired" stretching exercises are illustrated in Chapter 13.

*The editor is grateful to James Zuckermandel for his assistance in writing this chapter.

Table 30-1. Swimming overview

| BASIC SKILLS | MUSCLES INVOLVED |
|---|---|
| 1. Starts | Buttocks, lower back, quadriceps |
| 2. Turns | Buttocks, lower back, hamstrings, quadriceps |
| 3. Kicking | Buttocks, lower back, quadriceps |
| 4. Strokes | Latissimus dorsi, pectorals, deltoids, triceps, biceps, trapezius, abdominals |

PROBLEM AREAS:

Muscular fatigue
Stamina
Flexibility
Abdominals

AREAS TO EMPHASIZE:

- Develop the musculature involved in each specific stroke in order to prevent muscular fatigue.
- Utilize prolonged water work to develop cardiovascular fitness, interval training is an effective technique
- Emphasize flexibility exercises in order to maximize stroke efficiency and reduce the possibility of joint-related injuries
- Develop the abdominals as much as possible

Table 30-2. Off-season Swimming Nautilus Workout Program

| EXERCISE (in order) | PRIMARY MUSCLES DEVELOPED | SPECIFIC SKILLS INVOLVED |
|---|---|---|
| 1. Hip and Back | Buttocks, lower back | Starts, turns, kicks |
| 2. Leg Extension | Quadriceps | Starts, turns, kicks |
| 3. Leg Press | Buttocks, quadriceps | Starts, turns, kicks |
| 4. Leg Curl | Hamstrings | Starts, turns |
| 5. Pullover | Latissimus dorsi | All strokes |
| 6. Chinups | Latissimus dorsi, biceps | All strokes |
| 7. Double Chest (bent arm fly) | Pectorals | All strokes (primarily the breast stroke and the butterfly |
| 8. Dips | Pectorals, deltoids, triceps | All strokes |
| 9. Shrugs | Trapezius | All strokes |
| 10. Bentover Rowing | Teres major | All strokes |
| 11. Reverse Wrist Curls | Wrist extensors | All strokes |
| 12. Bent-leg Situps | Abdominals | All strokes |

- Perform 1 set of 8 to 12 reps of each exercise
- Take no more than 60 seconds to perform each set
- Rest no more than 30 seconds between each set
- To determine **total workout time:** multiply # of workouts by 1½ minutes, then subtract 30 seconds from total

*In-season only

Table 30-3. Off-season Swimming Universal Workout Program

| EXERCISE (in order) | PRIMARY MUSCLES DEVELOPED | SPECIFIC SKILLS INVOLVED |
|---|---|---|
| 1. Leg Press * | Buttocks, quadriceps | Starts, turns, kicks |
| 2. Leg Extension | Quadriceps | Starts, turns, kicks |
| 3. Leg Curl * | Hamstrings | Starts, turns |
| 4. Bench Press * | Pectorals, deltoids, triceps | All strokes |
| 5. Chinups * | Latissimus dorsi, biceps | All strokes |
| 7. Dips * | Pectorals, deltoids, | All strokes |
| 8. Shrugs * | Trapezius | All strokes |
| 9. Bentover Rowing | Teres major | All strokes |
| 10. Reverse Wrist Curls | Wrist extensors | All strokes |
| 11. Bent Leg Situps * | Abdominals | All strokes |

- Perform 1 set of 8 to 12 reps of each exercise
- Take no more than 60 seconds to perform each set
- Rest no more than 30 seconds between each set
- To determine **total workout time:** multiply # of workouts by 1½ minutes, then subtract 30 seconds from total

*In-season only

# CHAPTER 31
## Team Handball

Team handball is a sport requiring high levels of both personal fitness and gross motor abilities. Combining many of the skills utilized in football and soccer, team handball players should possess stamina, muscular endurance, explosive power, and coordination. A properly organized conditioning program can improve *each* of these aspects.

The basic element in a conditioning program for team handball should be a general, overall muscular development program. Such a program should concentrate on the development of the muscles of the legs, shoulder girdle, upper back, and arms. A muscular fitness program for team handball should promote an increase in both strength and endurance. A higher level of strength will directly affect an athlete's performance *on* the field. Greater endurance will prevent (or delay) the onslaught of debilitating muscular fatigue. Such fatigue is a frequent by-product of the excessive demand on the team handball player.

Proper development of the musculature used to grip the ball should also be an important part of the conditioning program for team handball. Higher levels of grip strength not only improves the athlete's ability to hold onto the ball, but also to his aptitude for controlling and dribbling the ball. Such skills play a basic role during *all* phases of the game.

Stamina for team handball should be developed through an extensive program of aerobic conditioning. Fartlek, interval, and circuit training —in varying combinations—are excellent programs for developing stamina for team handball.

*The editor is grateful to Captain Earl Greer for his assistance in writing this chapter.

## Table 31-1. Team handball overview

| BASIC SKILLS | MUSCLES INVOLVED |
| --- | --- |
| 1. Running | Buttocks, lower back, quadriceps, hamstrings |
| 2. Checking | Buttocks, quadriceps, lower back |
| 3. Shooting | Pectorals, deltoids, triceps, biceps, forearm flexors, latissimus dorsi |
| 4. Passing | Pectorals, deltoids, triceps, biceps, latissimus dorsi, forearm flexors |

PROBLEM AREAS:

Muscular fatigue
Stamina
Shoulders
Arms
Knees

AREAS TO EMPHASIZE:

- Develop the musculature involved in team handball in order to prevent muscular fatigue
- Develop cardiovascular fitness for team handball by means of a combination of interval, circuit, and fartlek training
- Emphasize flexibility and joint stability in order to reduce the possibility of injuries

## Table 31-2. Off-season Team Handball Nautilus Workout Program

| EXERCISE (in order) | PRIMARY MUSCLES DEVELOPED | SPECIFIC SKILLS INVOLVED |
|---|---|---|
| 1. Leg Extension* | Quadriceps | Running, checking |
| 2. Leg Press* | Buttocks, quadriceps | Running, checking |
| 3. Hip and Back* | Buttocks, lower back | Running, checking |
| 4. Leg Curl* | Hamstrings | Running |
| 5. Double Chest (bent arm flex movement) | Pectorals | Passing, shooting, checking |
| 6. Dips* | Pectorals, deltoids, triceps | Passing, shooting, checking |
| 7. Pullover | Latissimus dorsi | Passing, checking, shooting |
| 8. Chinups* | Latissimus dorsi, biceps | Passing, checking, shooting |
| 9. Triceps Extension | Triceps | Passing, blocking, shooting |
| 10. Biceps Curls | Biceps | Passing, shooting, dribbling |
| 11. Wrist Curls* | Forearm flexors | Grip, wrist, control, passing, dribbling, shooting |

- Perform 1 set of 8 to 12 reps of each exercise
- Take no more than 60 seconds to perform each set
- Rest no more than 30 seconds between each set
- To determine **total workout time:** multiply # of workouts by 1½ minutes, then subtract 30 seconds from total

*In-season only

Table 31-3. Off-season Team Handball Universal Workout Program

| EXERCISE (in order) | PRIMARY MUSCLES DEVELOPED | SPECIFIC SKILLS INVOLVED |
|---|---|---|
| 1. Leg Press* | Buttocks, quadriceps | Running, checking |
| 2. Leg Extension* | Quadriceps | Running, checking |
| 3. Leg Curl* | Hamstrings | Running |
| 4. Bench Press* | Pectorals, deltoids, triceps | Passing, shooting, checking |
| 5. Chinups* | Latissimus dorsi, biceps | Passing, shooting, checking |
| 6. Seated Press* | Deltoids, triceps | Passing, checking, shooting |
| 7. Lat Pulldown | Latissimus dorsi, biceps | Passing, shooting, checking |
| 8. Triceps Extension | Triceps | Passing, shooting, checking |
| 9. Bicep Curls | Biceps | Passing, shooting, dribbling |
| 10. Wrist Curls | Forearm flexors | Grip, wrist control, passing, dribbling, shooting |

- Perform 1 set of 8 to 12 reps of each exercise
- Take no more than 60 seconds to perform each set
- Rest no more than 30 seconds between each set
- To determine **total workout time:** multiply # of workouts by 1½ minutes, then subtract 30 seconds from total

*In-season only

# CHAPTER 32
## Tennis

Tennis is a sport which demands a high level of speed of movement, explosive power, and muscular endurance. All of these attributes can be improved significantly by increasing the strength of the muscles used during a tennis match. Tennis enthusiasts at all levels of competition can, therefore, improve the caliber of their game by becoming involved in a properly organized muscular development program.

This program should place special emphasis on the development of the abdominal muscles, legs, shoulder girdle, upper back and arms. Increased strength in these areas will enable the athlete to run and make changes in direction faster, reach out for and vigorously return those hard to reach balls, and sustain a more intense level of play throughout a physically demanding five-set match. An increase in upper arm and forearm strength will improve racket preparation efficiency of the tennis player, as well as racket control on impact and during the follow through. In addition, well conditioned muscles help prevent the nagging injuries associated with power serves (lower back, shoulder, and abdominal strains) and the traumatic, vibrational jarring (tennis elbow) often sustained when hitting the ball.

*The editor is grateful to Paul Assiante, head coach of the USMA varsity tennis team, for his assistance in writing this chapter.

Table 32-1. Tennis overview

| BASIC SKILLS | MUSCLES INVOLVED |
|---|---|
| 1. Running | Buttocks, quadriceps, hamstrings |
| 2. Serve | Deltoids, triceps, biceps, latissimus dorsi, trapezius |
| 3. Forehand | Latissimus dorsi, biceps, triceps, forearm flexors |
| 4. Backhand | Triceps, biceps, deltoids, latissimus dorsi, forearm flexors |
| 5. Raquet control | Forearm flexors, triceps, biceps |

PROBLEM AREAS:

Muscular fatigue
Stamina
Tennis elbow
Lower back and shoulder injuries

AREAS TO EMPHASIZE:

- Develop stamina by means of a comprehensive running/interval program.

- Develop the musculature involved in the basic tennis skills

- Increase joint stability by developing musculature facilitating joint movement

## Table 32-2. Tennis Nautilus Workout Program*

| EXERCISE (in order) | PRIMARY MUSCLES DEVELOPED | SPECIFIC SKILLS INVOLVED |
|---|---|---|
| 1. Leg Extension | Quadriceps | Running, stopping, starting, changing direction |
| 2. Leg Press | Buttocks, quadriceps | Changing direction while moving, quick starts |
| 3. Hip and Back | Buttocks, lower back | Running, serving, prevents lower back strains |
| 4. Leg Curls | Hamstrings | Running backwards/sidewards, changing direction while moving |
| 5. Double Shoulder (lateral raise) | Deltoids | Overhead serve, forehead, back hand |
| 6. Double Shoulder (seated press) | Deltoids, triceps | Power serve, forehand, backhand |
| 7. Shrugs | Trapezius | Serve, smash |
| 8. Pullover | Latissimus dorsi | Serve, smash, forehand, backhand |
| 9. Biceps Curl | Biceps | Serve, forehand, backhand, help prevent tennis elbow |
| 10. Triceps Extension | Triceps | Hitting the ball, arm extension, follow-through raquet control |
| 11. Wrist Curl | Forearm flexors | Grip strength for raquet control, wrist control, forehand and backhand |
| 12. Bent-knee Situps | Abdominal muscles | Power serve, smash, volley |

- Perform 1 set of 8 to 12 reps of each exercise during off-season
- Take nomore than 60 seconds to perform each set
- Rest no more than 30 seconds between each set
- To determine **total workout time:** multiply # of workouts by 1½ minutes, then subtract 30 seconds from total.

*For most individuals, tennis is a year-around sport. The frequency of the workouts should be adjusted according to the specific situation.

## Table 32-3. Tennis Universal Workout Program*

| EXERCISE (in order) | PRIMARY MUSCLES DEVELOPED | SPECIFIC SKILLS INVOLVED |
|---|---|---|
| 1. Leg Press | Buttocks, quadriceps | Running, starting, stopping, changing direction |
| 2. Leg Extension | Quadriceps | Changing direction while moving, fast starts and stops |
| 3. Leg Curl | Hamstrings | Running backward, sideward, fast starts and stops |
| 4. Seated Press | Deltoids, triceps | Power serve, smash, forehand, backhand |
| 5. Upright rowing | Biceps, deltoids | Serve, smash, forehand, backhand |
| 6. Dips | Pectorals, deltoids, triceps | Serve, forehand, backhand, smash |
| 7. Lat Pulldown | Latissimus dorsi, biceps | Forehand, backhand, serve, smash |
| 8. Shrugs | Trapezius | Power serve, smash |
| 9. Biceps Curls | Biceps | Power serve, forehand, helps prevent tennis elbow |
| 10. Triceps Extension | Triceps | Hitting the ball, arm extension, follow through |
| 11. Wrist Curls | Forearm flexors | Grip strength for raquet control, wrist control |
| 12. Bent-knee Situps | Abdominal muscles | Power serve, smash, volley |

- Perform 1 set of 8 to 12 reps of each exercise during off-season
- Take no more than 60 seconds to perform each set
- Rest no more than 30 seconds between each set
- To determine **total workout time:** multiply # of workouts by 1½ minutes, then subtract 30 seconds from total

*For most individuals, tennis is a year-around sport. The frequency of the workouts should be adjusted according to the specific situation.

# CHAPTER 33
## Track and Field

Track and field is a multifaceted sport, encompassing many different events. Primarily comprised of events performed on an individual basis, track and field has seventeen separate activities—ranging from runs (short sprints and middle and long distance runs), hurdles (high and low hurdles at varying distances), to field events (throwing, jumping, and vaulting).

Although each of the separate track events has a unique requirement (dimension) which should be considered in developing a conditioning program for track and field, several program commonalities exist. For **all** track events, a high level of "overall fitness" is desireable. The specific requirement, however, for each aspect of fitness (muscular fitness, flexibility, cardiovascular fitness, and body composition) varies from event to event.

Strength, for example, has a more substantial role for athletes who participate in the throwing events than for athletes who run the hurdles. Similarly, cardiovascular fitness is essential for long distance runners, while having little effect on the high jumper. For all track events, high levels of both muscular endurance and flexibility are a must. Flexibility is particularly important for pole vaulters and high jumpers.

To be as successful as possible, track and field athletes, whatever their specialty, should train on a year around basis. Because a listing of the training programs for the numerous track and field events is beyond the scope of this text, the reader should refer to earlier Chapters for specific program suggestions. A weight training program designed to develop the musculature involved in both running and jumping is included in Tables 33-1 and 33-2.

*The editor is grateful to Captain Robert Hoffman for his assistance in writing this chapter.

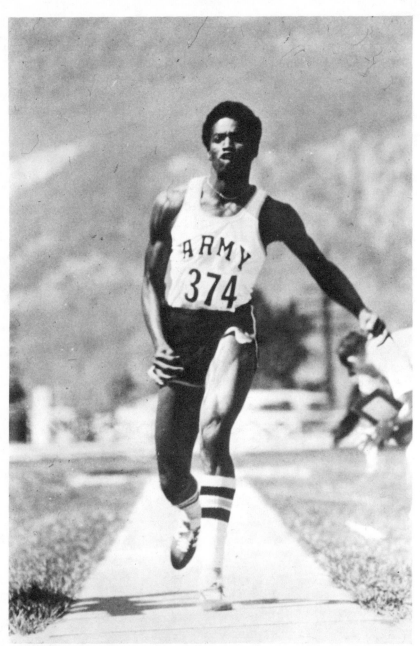

Muscular fitness is essential for **all** track events.

Table 33-1. Track and Field Universal Workout Program for
Running and Jumping

| EXERCISE (in order) | PRIMARY MUSCLES DEVELOPED | SPECIFIC SKILLS INVOLVED |
|---|---|---|
| 1. Leg Extension | Quadriceps | Running and jumping |
| 2. Leg Press | Buttocks, quadriceps | Running and jumping |
| 3. Hip and Back | Buttocks, lower back | Running and jumping |
| 4. Leg Curl | Hamstrings | Running |
| 5. Heel Riase | Calves | Running and jumping |
| 6. Pullovers | Latissimus dorsi | Stabilize the torso |
| 7. Shrugs | Trapezius | Stabilize the shoulder girdle |

- Perform 1 set of 8 to 12 reps of each exercise
- Take no more than 60 seconds to perform each set
- Rest no more than 30 seconds between each set
- To determine *total workout time:* multiply # of workouts by 1½ minutes, then subtract 30 seconds from total.

| EXERCISE (in order) | PRIMARY MUSCLES DEVELOPED | SPECIFIC SKILLS INVOLVED |
|---|---|---|
| 1. Leg Extension | Quadriceps | Running and jumping |
| 2. Leg Press | Buttocks, quadriceps | Running and jumping |
| 3. Leg Curl | Hamstrings | Running |
| 4. Heel Raise | Calves | Running and jumping |
| 5. Hyperextension | Lower back | Running and jumping |
| 6. Lat Pulldown | Latissimus dorsi | Stabilize the torso |
| 7. Shrugs | Trapezius | Stabilize the shoulder girdle |

- Perform 1 set of 8 to 12 reps of each exercise
- Take no more than 60 seconds to perform each set
- Rest no more than 30 seconds between each set
- To determine *total workout time:* multiply # of workouts by 1½ minutes, then subtract 30 seconds from total

Table 33-2. Track and Field Nautilus Workout Program for
Running and Jumping.

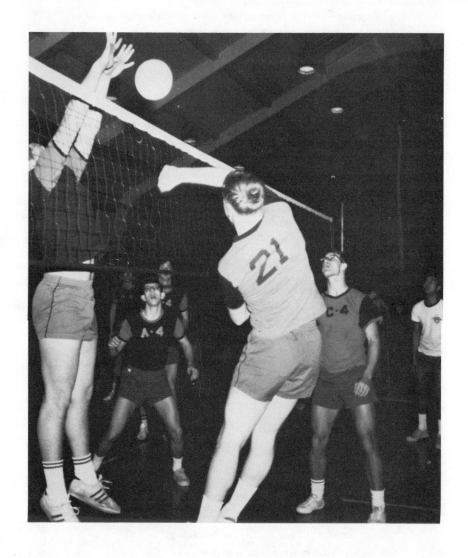

# CHAPTER 34
## Volleyball

Explosive power, endurance, flexibility and good motor abilities are all essentials of a successful volleyball player. A substantial increase in muscular fitness would improve each of the aforementioned factors and would also reduce the possibility of injuries common to volleyball players. Therefore, a properly organized muscular development training program is essential if the athlete hopes to reach his/her potential.

Competitive volleyball demands a very high level of both leg and shoulder girdle strength. An increased level of leg strength will permit the players to improve both vertical jump and speed of movement. Improved muscular fitness also enables the athlete to sustain his/her activity at a higher level of intensity for a much longer period of time.

An improvement in shoulder girdle strength and arm strength will result in an increase in a volleyballer's spiking and blocking efficiency. Such an improvement can also have a positive effect on a player's defensive abilities. The execution of the diving technique for defense, for example, requires this additional strength.

### JUMP TRAINING

The principle of **specificity of exercise** states that an athlete should duplicate, as nearly as possible, the sport movements under the conditions which the athlete will have to perform. Therefore, an athlete should jump to improve his/her jumping ability. A jump training program with weight training alone would be inadequate as weight training can only increase the athletes jump indirectly by developing strength in the appropriate muscle. The most effective conditioning program for improving jumping ability would combine both weight training and specificity jumping training.

In a specificity jump training program, the athlete should be concerned with quality jumps, not quantity without quality. Specificity jump training consists of two types of exercises: those which require maximum effort and those which duplicate as many relevant game conditions as possible. Every set of jumps should be done quickly with no hesitation between jumps. One variation that should be added is that one of the listed jumping exercises should be done while the athlete is either off balance or in transition between skill performances. Because

*The editor is grateful to Robert Bertucci, head coach of the USMA Volleyball Team, for his assistance in writing this chapter.

of the energy requirements of volleyball, jump training should consist of numerous bouts with a brief rest after each exercise. During a practice session, jump training should be interspersed throughout the practice. These training periods require maximal effort during performance. There should be 3 jump training periods per practice with 4 to 5 exercises per period. The periods should be scheduled at the beginning of practice, sometime during practice, and shortly after practice before the athlete cools down.

The exact exercises to be included in a jump training program are only limited by the athlete's imagination. Virtually any object which can be safely jumped over, off, on, in, or around can be employed in some aspect of jump training. Examples of jump training exercises include:

- **rope skipping** — the athlete executes a maximum jump on each skip until fatigued.
- **depth jumping** — the athlete jumps off a high object (e.g. bench) and immediately jumps back again in one motion.
- **jump reach** — the athlete jumps to touch a suspended object (e.g. rope) which is set a maximum jump height.
- **jump reach** — the athlete jumps to touch a suspended object (e.g. rope) which is set a maximum jump height.
- **jump slap** — partners jump up on opposite sides of the net and slap hands.

## FLEXIBILITY

Adequate flexibility is a prerequisite for successful volleyball. A high level of flexibility enhances muscular response, increases range of motion, and reduces the possibility of debilitating injuries. The volleyball skills most affected by a lack of flexibility are those involved with passing and receiving the ball. Such skills constitute almost 50% of the game of volleyball since they are required for backcourt play. The reader is referred to Chapter 13 for information on conditioning for flexibility.

## Table 34-1. Volleyball overview

| BASIC SKILLS | MUSCLES INVOLVED |
| --- | --- |
| 1. Running and jumping | Buttocks, quadriceps, hamstrings |
| 2. Serving | Deltoids, trapezius, latissimus dorsi |
| 3. Setting | Pectorals, deltoids, triceps, biceps |
| 4. Spiking | Deltoids, triceps, forearm flexors, latissimus dorsi |
| 5. Digging | Biceps, latissimus dorsi, trapezius, pectorals |
| 6. Blocking | Deltoids, latissimus dorsi, trapezius |

PROBLEM AREAS:

Muscular endurance
Stamina
Shoulder injuries
Leg muscle strains

AREAS TO EMPHASIZE:

- Use a comprehensive running/interval program to develop stamina
- Develop muscles identified as critical to performance of basic volleyball skills
- Emphasize flexibility conditioning
- Develop musculature of the shoulder girdle and legs
- Develop knee joint stability

## Table 34-2. Off-season Volleyball Nautilus Workout Program

| EXERCISE (in order) | PRIMARY MUSCLES DEVELOPED | SPECIFIC SKILLS INVOLVED |
|---|---|---|
| 1. Hip and Back* | Buttocks | Jumping, running |
| 2. Leg Extension* | Quadriceps | Jumping, running |
| 3. Leg Press | Buttocks, quadriceps | Jumping, running |
| 4. Leg Curl* | Hamstrings | Jumping, running |
| 5. Double Chest* (bent arm fly) | Pectorals | Setting, spiking |
| 6. Double Chest (decline press) | Pectorals, deltoids, | Setting, spiking, blocking |
| 7. Pullover* | Latissimus dorsi | Spiking |
| 8. Double Shoulder* (lateral raise) | Deltoids | Setting, spiking, blocking |
| 9. Double Shoulder* (seated press) | Deltoids, triceps | Setting, spiking |
| 10. Chin Ups* | Latissimus dorsi, biceps | Spiking, digging |
| 11. Wrist Curls* | Forearm flexors | Spiking, setting, wrist control |
| 12. Shrugs* | Trapezius | Serving, spiking, setting, blocking |

- Perform 1 set of 8 to 12 reps of each exercise during off-season
- Take no more than 60 seconds to perform each set
- Rest no more than 30 seconds between each set
- To determine **total workout time**: multiply # of workouts by 1½ minutes, then subtract 30 seconds from total

*In-season

# Volleyball

## Table 34-3. Off-season Volleyball Universal Workout Program

| EXERCISE (in order) | PRIMARY MUSCLES DEVELOPED | SPECIFIC SKILLS INVOLVED |
| --- | --- | --- |
| 1. Leg Press | Buttocks, quadriceps | Running, jumping |
| 2. Leg Extension* | Quadriceps | Running, jumping |
| 3. Leg Curl* | Hamstrings | Running |
| 4. Bench Press* | Pectorals, deltoids, triceps | Setting, spiking |
| 5. Chin Ups* | Latissimus dorsi, biceps | Spiking, digging, blocking |
| 6. Seated Press* | Deltoids, triceps | Spiking, setting, blockng |
| 7. Lat Pulldowns | Latissimus dorsi, biceps | Spiking |
| 8. Triceps Extension* | Triceps | Spiking |
| 9. Wrist Curls* | Forearm flexors | Spiking, setting, wrist control |
| 10. Shrugs* | Trapezius | Serving, spiking, setting, blocking |

- Perform 1 set of 8 to 12 reps of each exercise during off-season.
- Take no more than 60 seconds to perform each set
- Rest no more than 30 seconds between each set
- To determine **total workout time:** multiply # of workouts by 1½ minutes, then subtract 30 seconds from total
*In-season

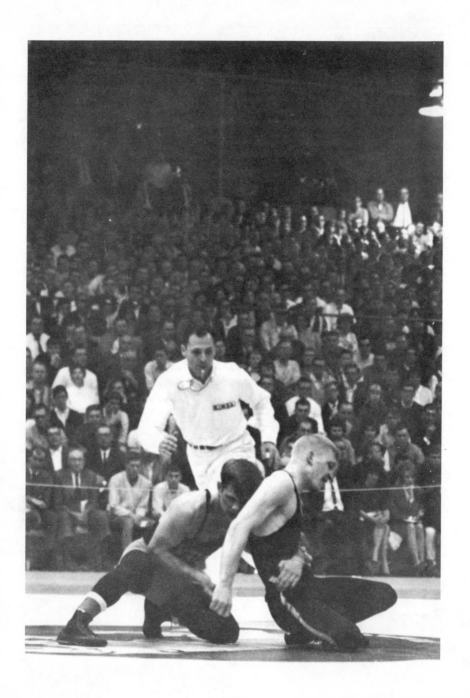

# CHAPTER 35
## Wrestling

Of all the sports popular in America today, wrestling is considered by many individuals to be the most strenuous and demanding athletic activity. A successful wrestler must have great explosive power, balance, speed, agility, flexibility and finesse. He must also be a good strategist when using or setting-up one of the many wrestling moves or holds he is required to learn through hours of devoted practice. It is also important that a wrestler be a staunch disciplinarian as far as his diet and training program are concerned. In addition, and probably most importantly, he must possess a very large amount of desire to win and the capability to bounce back if he doesn't...

Some of the foregoing attributes are inborn, but all can be developed by either the wrestler himself or with the help and guidance of a coach. The following muscular development program (Table 35-2, 35-3) has been scientifically developed specifically for the wrestler. By adopting this program and performing the exercises properly on a regular basis, phenomenal "sport-specific" strength can be developed resulting in greater success on the mat.

Wrestling actually involves all the major muscles of the body. Therefore, the recommended program includes exercises for each muscle group with special emphasis on the neck muscles and grip strength. During the wrestling season the program should be accomplished as indicated. (Some wrestlers abstain from strength training during the season for various reasons. This is counter productive in developing the championship caliber wrestler. A wrestler who does not at least participate in a *strength maintenance* program during the season will eventually lose some of his capability as a successful wrestler.)

*The editor is grateful to Al Rushatz for his assistance in writing this chapter.

## Table 35-1. Wrestling Overview

| BASIC SKILLS | MUSCLES INVOLVED |
|---|---|
| 1. Take downs (deep penetration) | Quadriceps, buttocks, deltoids, biceps |
| 2. Reversals (Switching power) | Deltoids, biceps, triceps |
| 3. Escapes (Explosive power) | Quadriceps, hamstrings, latissimus dorsi |
| 4. Control (Grip and leg strength) | Forearm flexors, deltoids, triceps, biceps, upper and lower leg |
| 5. Defense (Clearing power) | Deltoids, triceps, pectorals, biceps, forearm flexors, hamstrings, quadriceps |

PROBLEM AREAS:

> Muscular endurance
> Stamina
> Knee, shoulder, elbow and neck injuries
> Muscle pulls and strains

AREAS TO EMPHASIZE:

- Increase joint stability to protect against disabling injury
- Develop increased neck muscle strength for bridging, neck stabilization to resist nelsons, and prevent disabling injury
- Increase muscular endurance to sustain physical demands of an entire bout — especially during tournaments
- Develop increased grip strength, an extremely important attribute used in all phases of wrestling.
- Develop explosive power necessary to initiate moves from all positions
- Develop stamina by using a comprehensive running/interval program

## Table 35-2. Off-season Wrestling Nautilus Workout Program

| EXERCISE (in order) | PRIMARY MUSCLES DEVELOPED | SPECIFIC SKILLS INVOLVED |
|---|---|---|
| 1. Leg Extension | Quadriceps | Standup, switch, deep penetrations on takedowns, use of legs in cross body rides. |
| 2. Leg Press | Buttocks, quadriceps | Standup, switch, deep penetration on takedowns |
| 3. Hip and Back* | Buttocks, lower back | Defense against the cradle, standups, cross body ride |
| 4. Leg Curl* | Hamstrings | Clearning an ankle, defense against cradle |
| 5. Double Shoulder (lateral raise) | Deltoids | Overhook, extending the arms, switch, breakdowns |
| 6. Double Shoulder (seated press) | Deltoids, triceps | Breaking wrist tie-ups, arm extension, wrist rides, cradles |
| 7. Pullover | Latissimus dorsi | Underhooks, headlocks, double leg takedowns, overhead |
| 8. Chinups* | Latissimus dorsi, biceps | Tight waist rides, double leg takedowns, headlocks |
| 9. Dips* | Pectorals, deltoids, triceps | Recovering to all fours from the breakdown, initiating standups |
| 10. Biceps Curls | Biceps | Wrist rides, tight waists, ankle rides, initiate takedowns |
| 11. Wrist Curls | Forearm flexors | Wrist and ankle control, tight waist, arm tie ups |
| 12. Four Way Neck* | Neck muscles | Bridging, neck stabilization against nelsons, duck under takedowns |
| 13. Shrugs* | Trapezius | Bridging, neck stabilization, initiating takedowns |

- Perform 1 set of 8 to 12 reps of each exercise during off-season
- Take no more than 60 seconds to perform each set
- Rest no more than 30 seconds between each set
- To determine **total workout time:** multiply # of workouts by 1½ minutes, then subtract 30 seconds from total.

*In-season only

Wrestling

## Table 35-3. Off-season Wrestling Universal Workout Program

| EXERCISE (in order) | PRIMARY MUSCLES DEVELOPED | SPECIFIC SKILLS INVOLVED |
|---|---|---|
| 1. Leg Press* | Buttocks, quadriceps | Standup, switch, deep penetration on takedowns |
| 2. Leg Extension* | Quadriceps | Standup, switch, deep penetration on take-downs, leg rides |
| 3. Leg Curl* | Hamstrings | Clearing ankles, resisting cradles, initiating standups |
| 4. Bench Press* | Pectorals, deltoids, triceps | Overhook series, arm extension, cradles |
| 5. Chinups* | Latissimus dorsi, biceps | Tight waist, double leg takedowns, headlocks, tight waist |
| 6. Seated Press | Deltoids, triceps | Breakdowns, arm and leg control, tight waist, arm extensions |
| 7. Upright Rowing | Deltoids, biceps | Overhook, cross face, switch, breakdowns |
| 8. Hyperextensions | Lower back | Standups, breaking cradles, firemans carry series, takedowns |
| 9. Dips* | Pectorals, deltoids, triceps | Arm extension, recovering from breakdowns, initiating escapes |
| 10. Biceps Curls | Biceps | Tight waist, cross face, ankle rides, arm control |
| 11. Wrist Curls | Forearm flexors | Wrist and ankle control, cradles |
| 12. Neck Station* | Neck flexors, extensors | Bridging, neck stabilization against nelsons, duck under takedown series |
| 13. Shrugs* | Trapezius | Neck stabilization during bridging, against nelsons, takedowns |

- Perform 1 set of 8 to 12 reps of each exercise during off-season
- Take no more than 60 seconds to perform each set
- Rest no more than 30 seconds between each set
- To determine **total workout time:** multiply # of workouts by 1½ minutes, then subtract 30 seconds from total

*In-season only

## Table 35-4. Conditioning exercises for wrestling*

*For those wrestlers interested in variety in their conditioning program or those who do not have access to either Nautilus or Universal equipment, the following exercises are suggested to compliment both pre-season and in-season training.

**1. Rope Climbing** — A 1½-2 inch hemp or cotton rope should be used for this exercise. The rope should be hung from the ceiling of the wrestling room when possible in order to make it readily available to team members and provide padded floor protection. Rope climbing is an exceptionally good exercise which is "wrestling specific" as far as strength development is concerned. This exercise is initiated from the sitting position on the floor or mat with legs astride the rope, and hands grasping the rope about 6 inches above eye level. The wrestler should proceed to climb up the rope hand over, as far as he can, using his hands only. If he reaches the top of the rope he should return down the rope to the starting position, again without the use of his legs. If, during any part of the exercise, the legs are needed to keep his progress going the wrestler should use them to complete the exercise (climb to the top and return). However, the goal to be kept in mind is to climb to the top of the rope and return to the starting position without the use of the legs.

**2. Rope Jumping** — This exercise is used to provide limited stress on the cardiovascular system (heart and lungs) but more importantly develop smooth foot-work and general agility while in the standing or up position. Using both single and double foot jumps, the wrestler should start by endeavoring to jump rope for 5 minutes without stopping. Progress will be indicated by longer periods of sustained rope jumping (up to 10 minutes) and an increase of jumps or skips per minute.

**3. Pullups** — Pullups are accomplished by grasping an overhead bar with the palms of the hand facing away from you. Both the positive (up) and negative (down) parts of this exercise should be performed slowly and deliberately. If the wrestler can not do 12 pullups he should do as many as he can, then, with the aid of a chair or stool, do the negative portion of the exercise (slowly) until 12 repetitions are performed. If the wrestler can do more than 12 pullups he should use his jump rope to tie the weight plate around his waist which will limit him to 12 pullups.

**4. Pipe Twisters** — For this exercise the wrestler should use a piece of pipe or wooden pole (approximately 2 inches in diameter), 18 inches long with a ¼ inch hole drilled through the middle. To assemble the "pipe twister" the wrestler should push one end of his jump rope through the ¼ inch hole and tie a knot in the rope large enough to prevent the rope from sliding back through the hole. Using the other end of the rope, tie an adequate amount of weight plates to allow for a 60 second exercise. To perform this exercise the wrestler should hold the pipe about chin level with arms parallel to the floor and slowly twist the pipe, raising the weight Plate(s) from the floor to the pipe. When the weight touches the pipe the twisting action should be reversed and the weight slowly lowered to the floor. (If the weight used does not permit the wrestler to keep his arms parallel with the floor he should support them with the back of a chair, a bookshelf, etc. This exercise is excellent for grip strength development.

**5. Bridging with Weights** — This exercise is designed to increase the wrestler's bridging capability. Again, in order to afford sufficient stress to increase strength, this exercise will consist of normal back bridging with the addition of a plate weight held on the wrestler's chest. This exercise is accomplished by laying flat on the floor with a weight commensurate with the level of the wrestler's strength development held on the chest and then, executing a back bridge, raise the chest as high as possible. When a maximum height bridge is attained the wrestler will lift the plate from his chest, and, with arms straight, try to touch the plate to the floor behind his head and then return it to his chest and return to the starting position. (If mats are not readily available to protect the head during the bridge a folded towel should suffice.)

**6. Dynamic Neck Exercise** — This exercise develops strength in the neck muscles and, just as important, insures that maximum flexibility of the neck is maintained. This exercise requires the help of a fellow wrestler to provide the resistance needed to increase neck strength. The wrestler accomplishes the exercise by laying on his back on a press bench, etc., with his shoulders even with the edge of the bench (head and neck unsupported) and, with his partner providing resistance to his movements by holding his head, he raises, lowers and moves his head side to side. This exercise should be done until muscles are sufficiently fatigued.

**Running** — Running is mentioned here to remind the wrestler that running is a "must" for any program designed to help improve performance on the mat. As mentioned earlier in this book, the cardio-respiratory system of your body (heart, lungs, and circulation network) is what gets the oxygen from the surrounding atmosphere you perform in to your muscles and at the same time carries the by-products of energy production (carbon dioxide, etc.) to the lungs for expulsion from the body. Basically, the efficiency with which this system transports these gases determines your staying power or stamina on the mat. If you "run out of gas" on the mat it's because your transport system has let you down. This system, much like your skeletal muscles, responds to stress by getting stronger or more efficient. Therefore, when you run and stress your cardio-respiratory system it responds by becoming more efficient and affords you more staying power on the mat. Just as your routine for strength development of the skeletal muscles is sport, specific, your running program should be sport specific. That is to say, it should be made up of prolonged submaximal effort running (aerobic) as well as short maximal effort sprinting (anaerobic). Your skeletal muscle can be very highly developed but, without a very efficient transport system to get oxygen to them, they will not be able to sustain you through an entire wrestling match. Run with mat performance in mind — every day.

The foregoing strength training program, as any program concerned with personal development, requires a good amount of dedication, desire, fortitude on the part of the individual concerned with improving capabilities. Another "important" ingredient in any such program is consistency. Unfortunately, consistency can breed boredom. Therefore, there will be days when the last thing you will feel like doing is engaging in your strength training routine. This is where the dedication and desire come in. It's the easiest thing in the world to find an excuse why you can't make it to a workout a certain day. But, if you make up your mind that your workout is a **necessary** part of your daily routine, just like eating and sleeping are, you **will** find the time and drive needed to complete your workout. A winner finds a way to do it — a loser finds an excuse.